CHAIR YOGA

— FOR —

WEIGHT LOSS

15-Minute Daily Exercises for
Seniors Over 60
to Boost Strength, Flexibility,
and Shed Pounds –
Look and Feel Younger in Just 28 Days!

RICHARD LANE

Before you go any further,
Download Your FREE 28 DAY Chair Workout Challenge Plan Now!

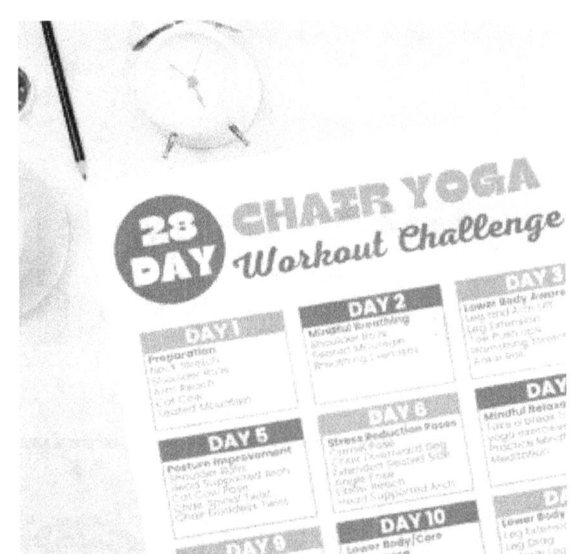

As a way of saying

"Thank You"

for your interest in our book, we would like to gift you this exercise chart **100% FREE!**

Go to:

http://idea2book.com/richardlane/chairyoga

*This is a limited time offer and can expire at any time.

Table of Contents

Introduction   5

What is Chair Yoga?   7

Chair Yoga Benefits for Seniors   8

Why a 28-Day Challenge?   10

Preparing for The 28-Day Challenge   11

The 28-Day Challenge   13

    WEEK 1   14

       Day 1: Preparation   14

       Day 2: Mindful Breathing   21

       Day 3: Lower Body Awareness   23

       Day 4: Upper Body Awareness   28

       Day 5: Posture Improvement   34

       Day 6: Relaxation/Stress Reduction Poses   37

       Day 7: Mindful Relaxation   42

    WEEK 2   43

       Day 8: Lower Body Strength   43

       Day 9: Core Strength   49

       Day 10: Lower Body/Core Endurance   51

       Day 11: Lower Body Strength   56

       Day 12: Core Strength   57

       Day 13: Isometric Strength   58

       Day 14: Active Recovery   62

    WEEK 3   63

       Day 15: Upper Body Strength   63

       Day 16: Lower Body Strength   68

       Day 17: Core Strength   69

Day 18: Spinal Health   72

Day 19: Upper Body Strength   75

Day 20: Hip Mobility   78

Day 21: Active Recovery   80

WEEK 4   81

Day 22: Functional Movement 1   81

Day 23: Functional Movement 2   87

Day 24: Upper Body Strength   91

Day 25: Functional Movement 1   92

Day 26: Core Strength   93

Day 27: Lower Body Strength   94

Day 28: Culmination   95

Bonus Section 1: Healthy Meal Plan for Seniors Over 60   99

Breakfast   99

Morning Snack   100

Lunch   100

Afternoon Snack   101

Dinner   101

Evening Snack   102

Wrap-Up   102

Bonus Section 2: Healthy Habits for Weight Loss and Overall Health   103

#1: Establish a Bedtime Routine   103

#2: Eat Whole Food   104

#3: Practice Stress Release Habits   104

#4: Drink 2.25 Liters of Water Daily   104

#5: Eat More Slowly   104

#6: Lift Weights to Lose Weight   105

#7: Fill Up on Fiber   106

#8: Meal Prep   106

Conclusion   107

Introduction

We all know we must exercise to improve our health, fitness, and overall well-being. Yet, as a senior, that advice can be pretty frustrating. After all, you don't have the mobility, flexibility, and strength you once had. Your get-up-and-go may have gotten up and left long ago, and your back may go out more than you do.

As a result of these realities, you can't do many of the exercise and fitness routines out there. You may be unable to run, jump, skip, or do calisthenics. But that doesn't mean you cannot exercise effectively and safely at your level.

How?

With Chair Yoga.

Chair yoga has become extremely popular recently as more and more seniors discover just how good a fit it is for them. Yet, this is no passing fad. Using a chair to make yoga movements more accessible to seniors and others with mobility challenges has been done for decades.

Over the years, older people worldwide have been using this form of exercise to lose weight, strengthen their muscles, increase mobility and balance, boost their circulation and heart health, and improve their posture.

Now it's your turn.

This 28-day chair yoga challenge is ideal for introducing the chair yoga exercise habit into your life. Over a month, you will gradually introduce chair yoga movements into your daily schedule in a non-threatening and accessible way. Each day, you'll add slightly more challenging exercises, requiring your body to progressively adapt by getting stronger and more flexible.

The end of the 28-day challenge is just the start of your chair yoga journey. You will have introduced chair yoga as part of your life habits. Your month of chair exercise will have produced a stronger, healthier, leaner, more balanced body so that you'll be more able to pursue a vibrant, independent life.

And you won't want to stop.

What is Chair Yoga?

Chair yoga is a modified form of yoga in which one either sits on a chair or uses a chair as a balance support when performing yoga movements.

Many people lack the mobility required to constantly get up and down from the floor during regular yoga poses. Chair yoga allows you to reap the benefits of yoga exercise while remaining in a stable, safe position.

Performing yoga exercises while seated helps you to remain relaxed. Relaxation helps synchronize your movements with your breathing, a fundamental part of yoga practice.

The critical characteristics of chair yoga are:

- Accessibility
- Adaptability
- Maintaining Balance
- Stability
- Versatility
- Breathing Focus

Chair Yoga Benefits for Seniors

The chair replaces a yoga mat as the main prop used in chair yoga. As such, it becomes an extension of the body, opening the benefits of yoga to people with mobility issues, joint problems, and nagging pain that prevents them from getting up and down from the floor.

Here are six benefits you'll receive when you make chair yoga part of your life:

1. Strength Improvement

Many chair yoga exercises involve moving your muscles through their full range of movement or holding them in an isometric hold position. This places adaptive stress on the muscle. Your body has a built-in stress adaptation mechanism by which your muscles respond by getting slightly bigger and stronger. Adapting allows the muscles to meet the stress better next time.

The stronger your muscles, the more stable you will be on your feet. This is especially true for your lower body muscles, such as the quadriceps, glutes, hamstrings, and calves. You will have a solid, stable base when these muscles are strong. This will help you move confidently and recover if you slip without tumbling over.

2. Enhanced Balance

As well as increasing strength, chair yoga promotes your balance by improving your body's proprioception. This is your ability to sense where your arms and legs are in space without looking at them. The greater your proprioception, the less likely you'll suffer from a fall.

Yoga involves many balance-enhancing movements. Using a chair makes these exercises accessible to seniors and others who would otherwise be unable to do them.

3. Greater Flexibility

As we age, we steadily lose flexibility. Chair yoga gently and gradually counters this age-related loss, helping you regain the range of movement you need to live a productive, independent life.

Chair yoga poses allow you to lengthen and elongate your muscles safely, reducing the risk of injury. You'll also be performing gentle rotation movements that promote joint mobility.

4. Weight Loss

People with limited mobility cannot do many traditional weight loss exercises like running or using a rowing machine. Chair yoga provides an accessible alternative to help them burn calories and lose body fat.

Chair yoga will not burn as many calories as running. Still, if accompanied by a daily caloric deficit, it will allow for a steady energy burn that will help you lose weight safely and permanently.

5. Improved Heart Health

The gentle, flowing movements involved in chair yoga boost circulation. As a result, the oxygen-rich blood supply to your muscles speeds up, improving muscle function.

Blood pressure is a significant heart health marker. Several chair yoga exercises are specifically designed to lower blood pressure and strengthen the heart. Unlike many cardio exercise options, chair yoga allows you to improve your cardio fitness without elevating your heart rate to an unsafe level.

6. Greater Independence

The improved strength, flexibility, and balance resulting from regular chair yoga practice will make it much easier to perform daily tasks like reaching, bending, and standing. As a result, tasks like carrying groceries, vacuuming, and walking up and down stairs will be more manageable for you.

Chair yoga will also make you far more confident on your feet. Your fear of falling will be greatly reduced, and your confidence in doing things you thought were beyond your limits will increase.

Chair yoga will enhance your emotional well-being. Your stress level will be reduced, and you will be a calmer, more relaxed person. You'll also be empowered to maintain a positive outlook and approach daily challenges with resilience and independence.

Why a 28-Day Challenge?

Undertaking a 28-day challenge can be an empowering journey toward improved physical and mental well-being. Research shows that forming a new habit takes between 21 and 28 days. When you commit to a 28-day challenge, you can implement a consistent yoga practice that will become ingrained in your daily routine.

Consistency is vital to experiencing the full benefits of chair yoga, including increased flexibility, strength, and relaxation. By committing to a structured, progressive daily plan over 28 days, you will see daily progress in your physical abilities and mental clarity.

Every day, you will have an opportunity to build upon your established foundation. The 28-day challenge also encourages you to be present in each moment, paying attention to your breath, body sensations, and thoughts during your session.

A 28-day timeframe provides a clear and achievable goal for you to work towards. Breaking the challenge into manageable daily sessions makes it less overwhelming and more attainable. As a result, you'll be more motivated to stay committed and engaged throughout the challenge.

By the end of the 28-day challenge, you will feel more confident and comfortable with your yoga routine. This will make it easier to continue practicing beyond the initial 28 days and integrate chair yoga into your lifestyle for ongoing health and well-being.

Preparing for The 28-Day Challenge

The success of your 28-day chair yoga challenge depends largely upon thoughtful preparation. Here are half a dozen essential steps to take before starting the challenge:

1. Consult with Your Healthcare Provider

Before beginning the challenge, you should consult with your primary healthcare provider. This is especially important if you have any underlying health conditions or limitations. I recommend taking a copy of this book to show your doctor precisely what the challenge involves.

2. Set Clear Goals

Think realistically about the goals you want to achieve from the 28-day challenge. Foremost among these should be establishing chair yoga as a lifestyle habit. You should also set realistic, measurable goals for improving your strength, flexibility, balance, confidence, and mobility.

Clarifying your objectives will help you stay focused and motivated throughout the challenge.

3. Find a Sturdy Chair

The main piece of equipment required for the challenge is a sturdy chair. You should use the same chair every day. Here are the requirements for a good exercise chair:

- Sturdy base
- Not overly padded
- Backrest
- Armrests

Do not use a chair that has rollers or that otherwise moves around. If you use a wheelchair, ensure you put the brakes on before starting.

4. Create a Dedicated Space

Find a quiet and comfortable space in your home to practice chair yoga without distractions. Your chair should have at least three feet of clear space around it to allow unrestricted movement.

5. Schedule Your Sessions

Block out dedicated time in your daily schedule for your chair yoga practice. Whether you prefer to practice in the morning to energize your day or in the evening to unwind and relax, establishing a consistent practice time will help you prioritize your commitment to the challenge.

The 28-Day Challenge

Your 28-day chair yoga challenge involves a gradual progression whereby you challenge your body in increasingly difficult ways as the days go by. In Week One, you will build the program's foundation and familiarize yourself with several critical poses focused on improving posture and stability. You'll also learn how to breathe to enhance your movement and how to develop mindfulness as you engage in your chair yoga sessions.

DAY 01 Preparation

Sit upright in your chair, with your feet firmly planted on the floor and your hands resting on your thighs, palms down. Take a deep breath through your nose as you pull your shoulder blades back and down and open your chest.

Take five deep breaths, releasing the air through your nose. Feel your body relaxing and the tension leaving your body with each exhalation.

EXERCISE 01
NECK STRETCH

1. Sit tall with your spine erect and your feet flat on the floor. Rest your hands on your thighs or in your lap. Allow your shoulders to relax down away from your ears. Feel the natural lengthening of your spine.

2. Place your right hand on your head, fingers just above your left ear. Slowly tilt your head to the right, bringing your ear toward your shoulder. Apply gentle pressure with your hand.

3. Avoid lifting or lowering the shoulder; focus on the gentle stretch along the side of your neck.

4. Hold the position for fifteen seconds, feeling a comfortable stretch. You should feel a gentle pull along the opposite side of your neck. Slowly bring your head back to the center, maintaining an upright posture.

5. Repeat on the opposite side.

6. Complete three repetitions on each side.

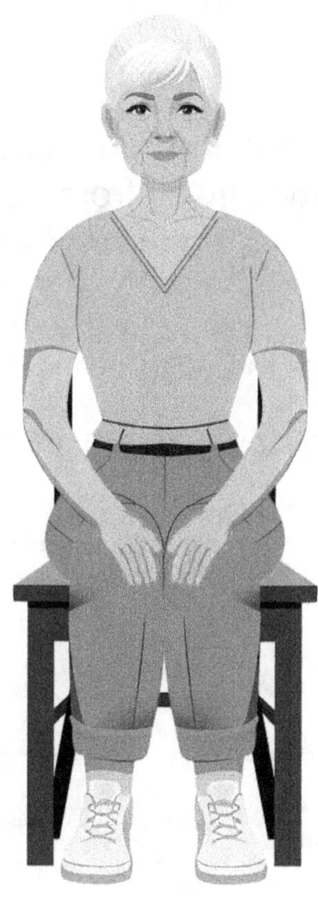

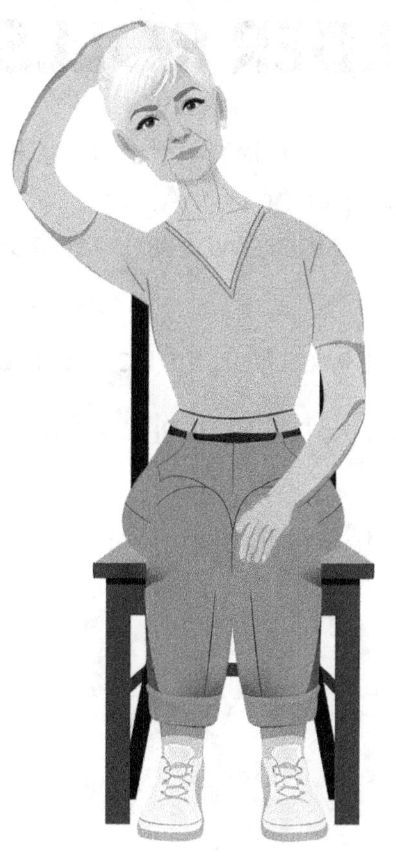

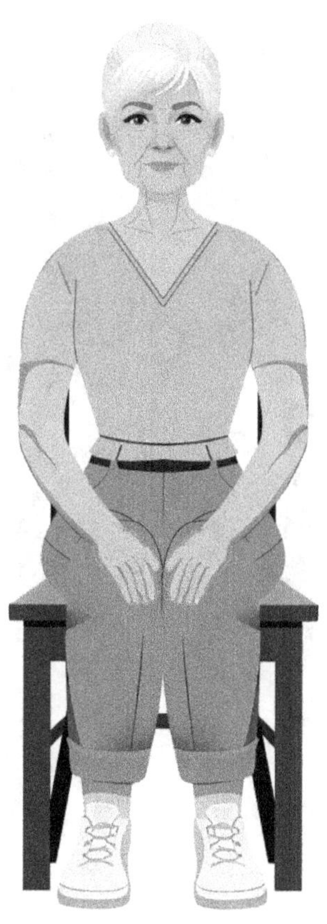

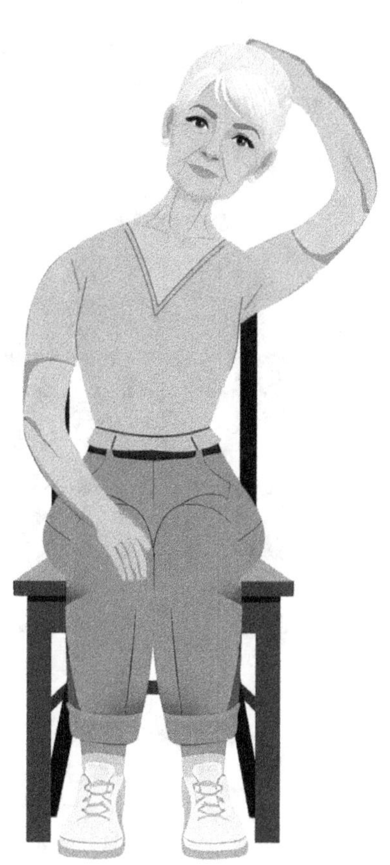

EXERCISE 02
SHOULDER ROLLS

1. Sit with your feet flat on the floor. Ensure your back is straight and your hands are resting on your thighs or lap. Allow your shoulders to relax down, away from your ears. Find a neutral position where your spine is aligned, and there's no unnecessary shoulder tension.

2. Inhale deeply as you lift both shoulders toward your ears in a smooth, circular motion.

3. Exhale as you roll your shoulders forward, bringing them down and around in a circular motion.

4. Complete ten repetitions.

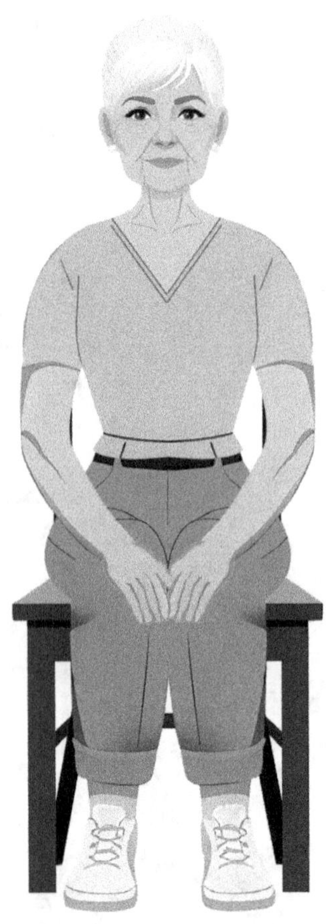
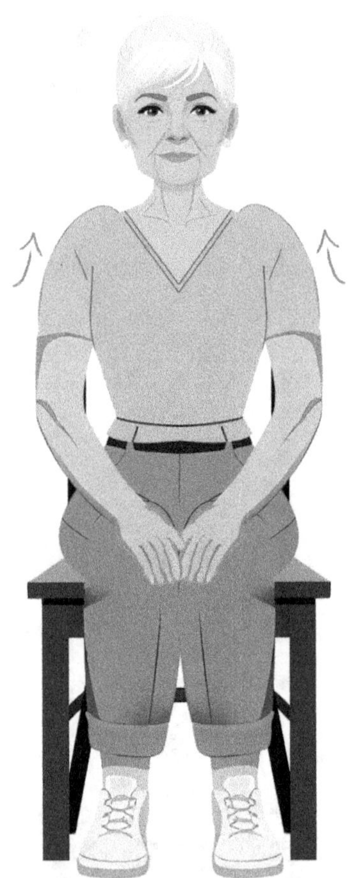

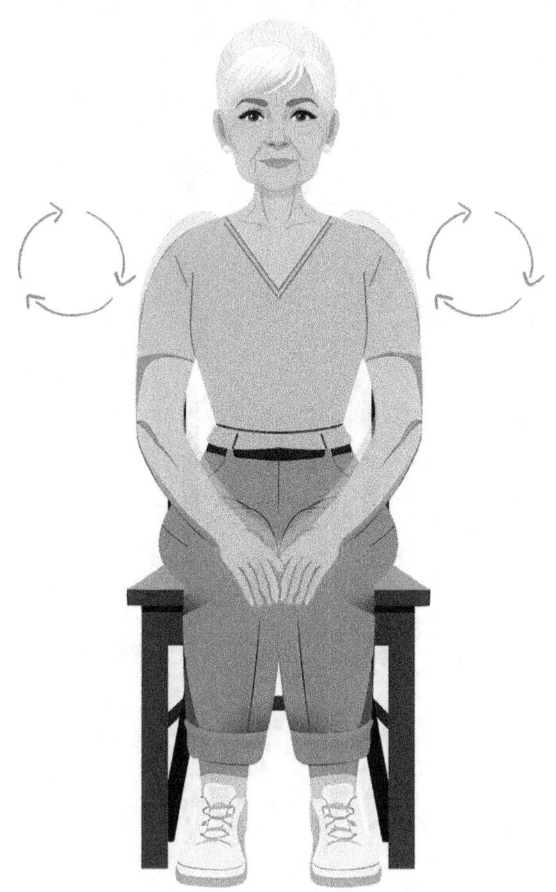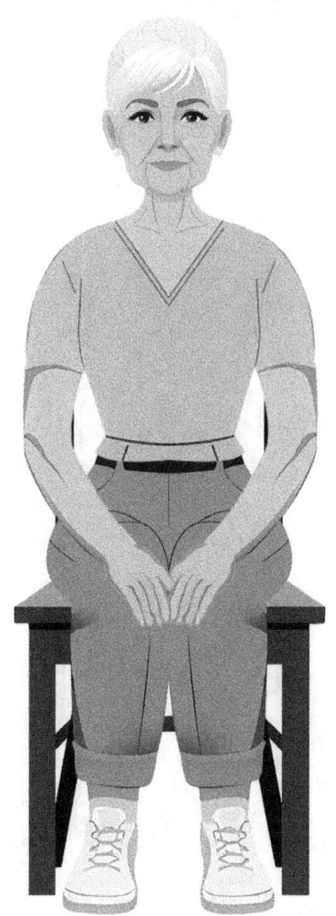

EXERCISE 03
ARM REACH

1. Sit upright with your feet flat on the floor and your hands resting on your thighs.

2. With your shoulder blades pulled back, inhale deeply through your nose as you raise both arms overhead and reach toward the ceiling.

3. Hold the extended reach for a count of three, feeling the stretch through your arms and back.

4. Lower your arms to the start position.

5. Complete five repetitions.

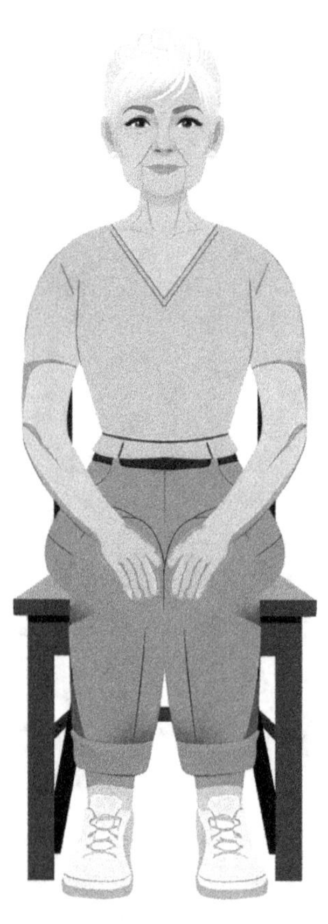

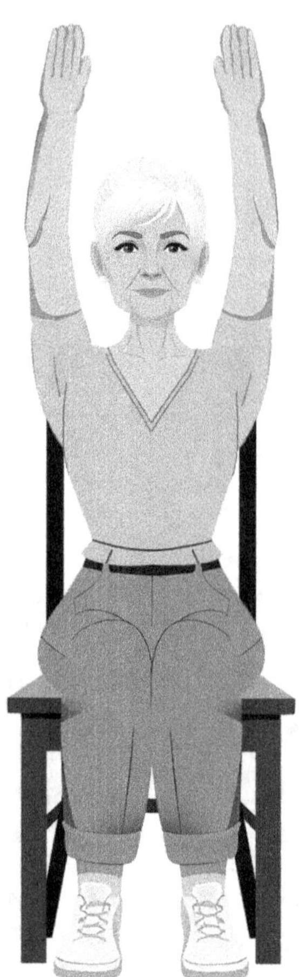

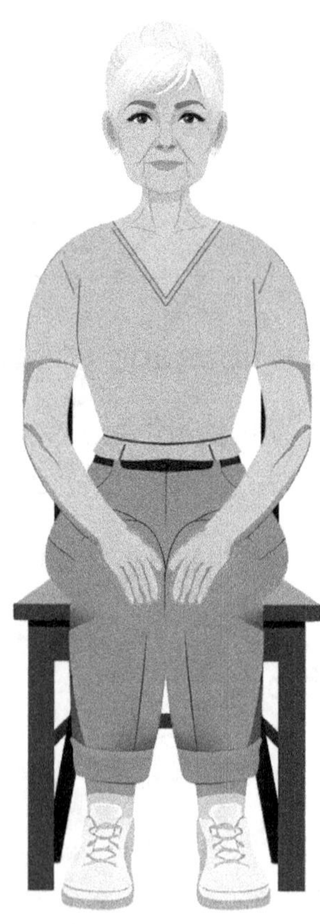

EXERCISE 4
CAT COW

1. Sit on a chair with your feet flat on the floor and your back straight. Place your hands on your knees or thighs.

2. Inhale and arch your back, lifting your chest (cow pose).

3. As you exhale, round your back, tuck your chin to your chest, and draw your navel in (cat pose).

4. Continue to flow between cow and cat poses with your breath, inhaling for the cow and exhaling for the cat.

5. Perform ten repetitions, feeling the stretch and release in your spine.

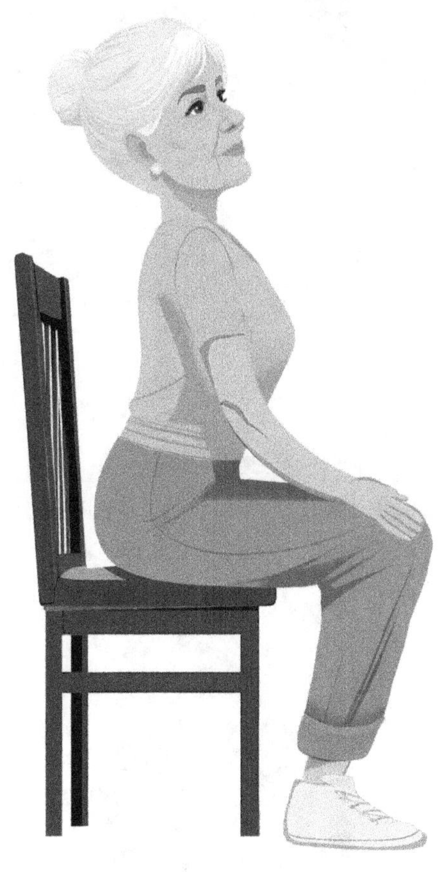 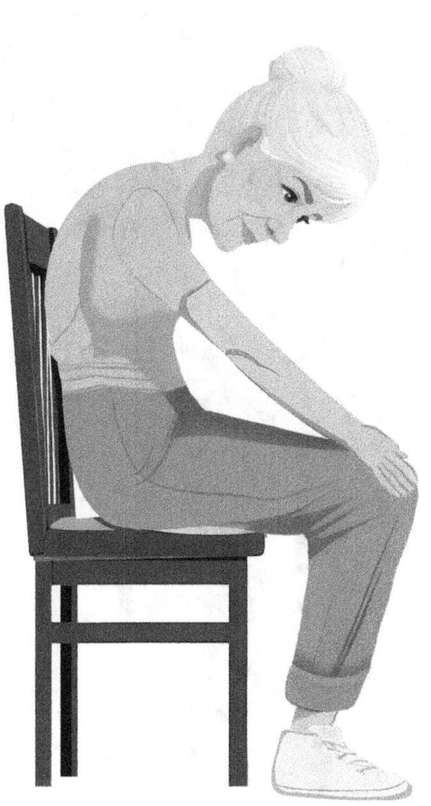

EXERCISE 5
SEATED MOUNTAIN

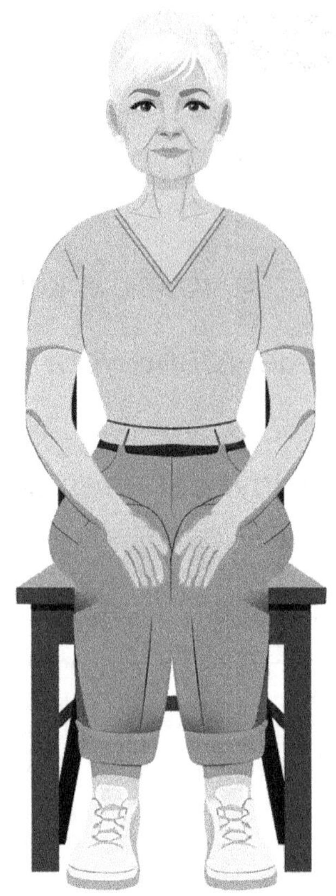

1. Sit tall with your hands resting on your thighs and feet firmly planted on the floor.

2. Breathe in as you raise your arms overhead. Interlock your fingers in the extended arm position.3. Push toward the ceiling as you extend your spine upward.

3. Breathe out as you return to the start position.

4. Perform ten repetitions of this exercise.

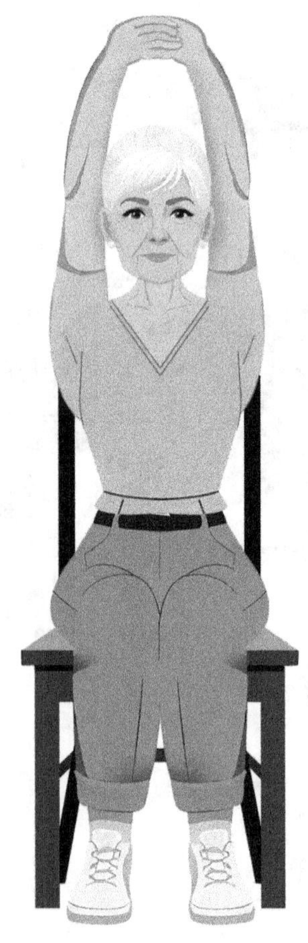

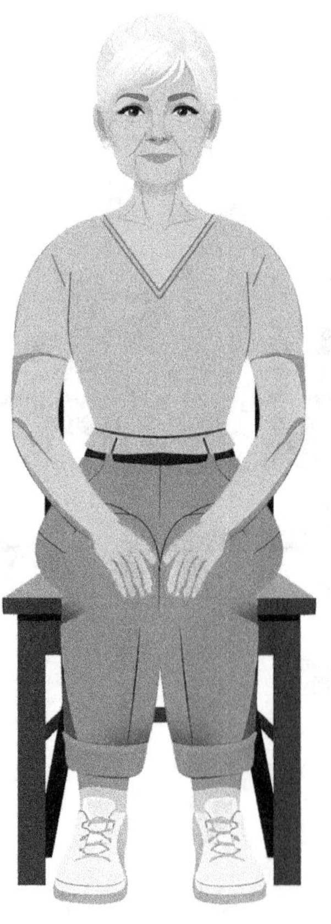

DAY 02 Mindful Breathing

Sit upright in your chair, with your feet firmly planted on the floor and your hands resting on your thighs, palms down. Take a deep breath through your nose as you pull your shoulder blades back and down and open your chest.

Take five deep repetitions, releasing the air through your nose. Feel your body relaxing and the tension leaving your body with each exhalation.

EXERCISE 1
SHOULDER ROLLS

Complete ten repetitions.

EXERCISE 2
SEATED MOUNTAIN

Do this exercise for ten reps.

You will now focus on your breathing using a couple of yoga-inspired techniques to enhance your muscle-mind connection, calm your mind, and release bodily tension. You will perform these breathing exercises while sitting in your chair.

Deep nasal breathing is the most effective way to produce a relaxed, calm state. When you draw in air through the nasal passage, you can achieve a greater oxygen intake into the bloodstream.

When you breathe through the nose, your breathing rate naturally slows down, producing a calmer state. As a result, your mind starts to relax. It's as if a switch is triggered to counter stress.

Breathing through the nose is not natural. For it to become habitual, we need to work at it.

Begin by drawing in deep nasal breaths for 30 seconds every minute. Build this up so that you're breathing through your nose for a minute at a time. Continue until you are breathing nasally for 5 minutes at a time.

Stand or sit comfortably. Now, take a long, deep breath through your nose until your lungs are full and your chest is inflated. Hold this breath for five full seconds. Then, allow the breath to leave your body slowly.

Consider expanding and compressing the diaphragm as an accordion on every inward and outward breath.

When you are breathing optimally, you will take in no more than ten breaths a minute, ideally just seven or eight. Your goal is to achieve as many sub-10 breath minutes as possible in your day.

BREATHING EXERCISE

1. Get comfortable, either standing or sitting.

2. Breathe in through the nose for 5 seconds. Feel your stomach pushing out as the energy-giving oxygen fills your lungs.

3. Hold for 20 seconds. Feel the oxygen circulating around your body as it gives life to your trillions of cells.

4. Repeat this process four more times.

Practice deep nasal breathing for the remainder of the 28-day challenge.

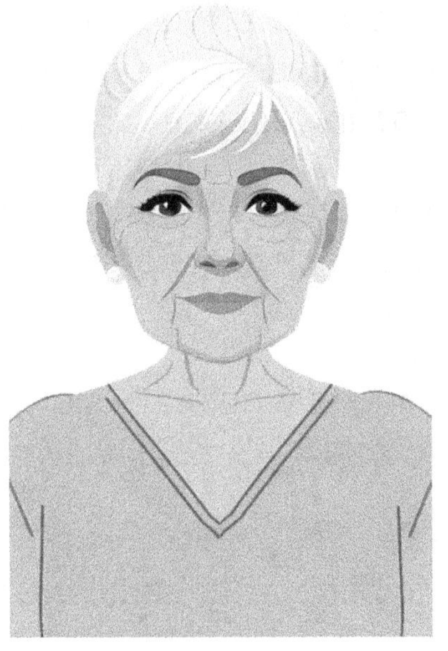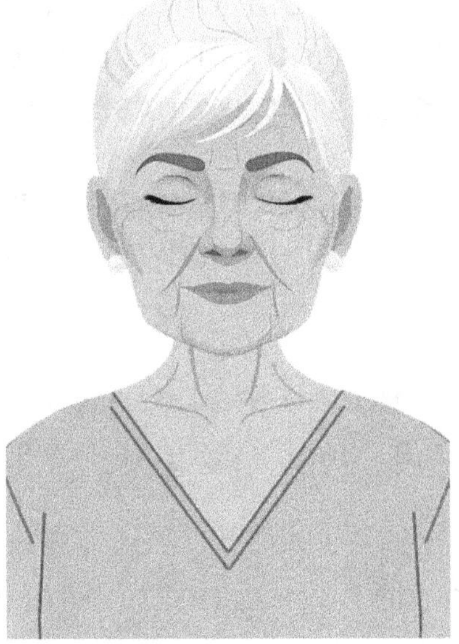

DAY 03 Lower Body Awareness

EXERCISE 1
LEG & ARM LIFT

1. Sit with your back straight and your feet flat on the floor, hip-width apart. Relax your shoulders and place your hands on your knees.

2. Inhale as you lift your right arm forward and up to shoulder height. Keep your palm facing upward.

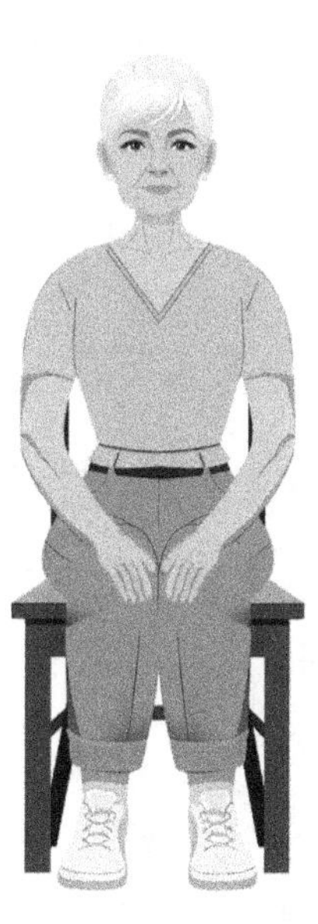 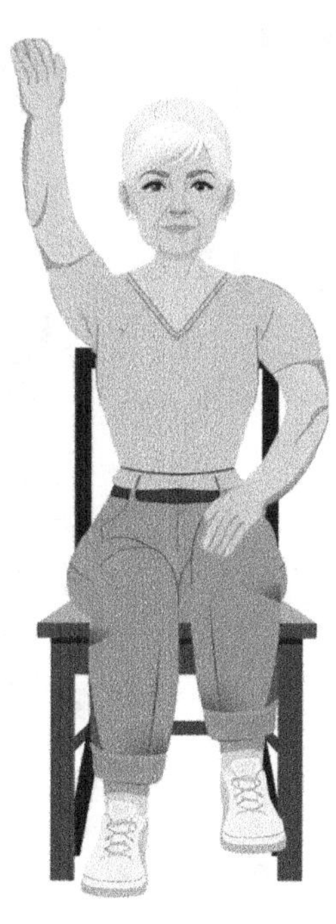 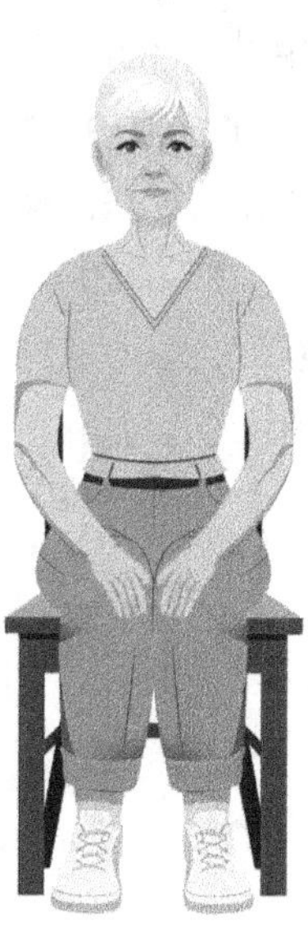

3. Simultaneously lift your left foot off the ground by about twelve inches.

4. Hold the raised arm and leg position for five seconds, maintaining your balance. Focus on a point in front of you to help with stability.

5. Repeat with the opposite arm and leg.

6. Do this exercise ten times.

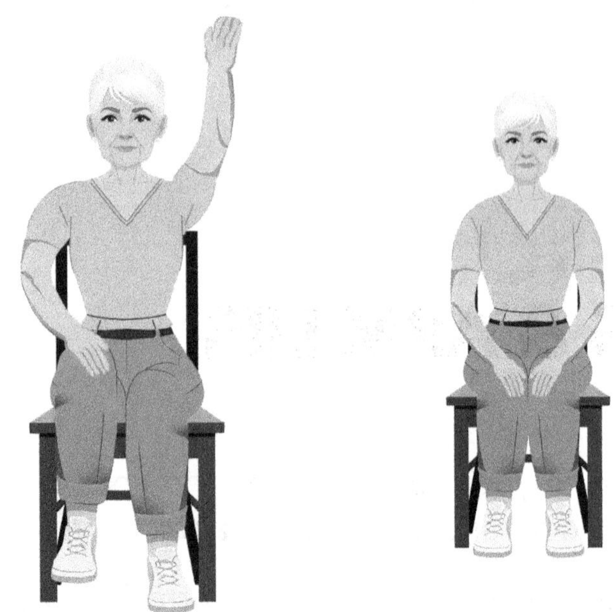

EXERCISE 2
LEG EXTENSION

1. Sit upright with your shoulder pulled back and chest out. Place your hands on the chair arms for support. Your legs should be bent at right angles, and your feet should be firmly planted on the floor.

2. Straighten out your right leg until it is just short of full extension. Hold for a five-second count as you flex the muscles in your quadriceps.

3. Slowly return your leg to its original position.

4. Repeat for ten repetitions.

5. Do the same with the left leg.

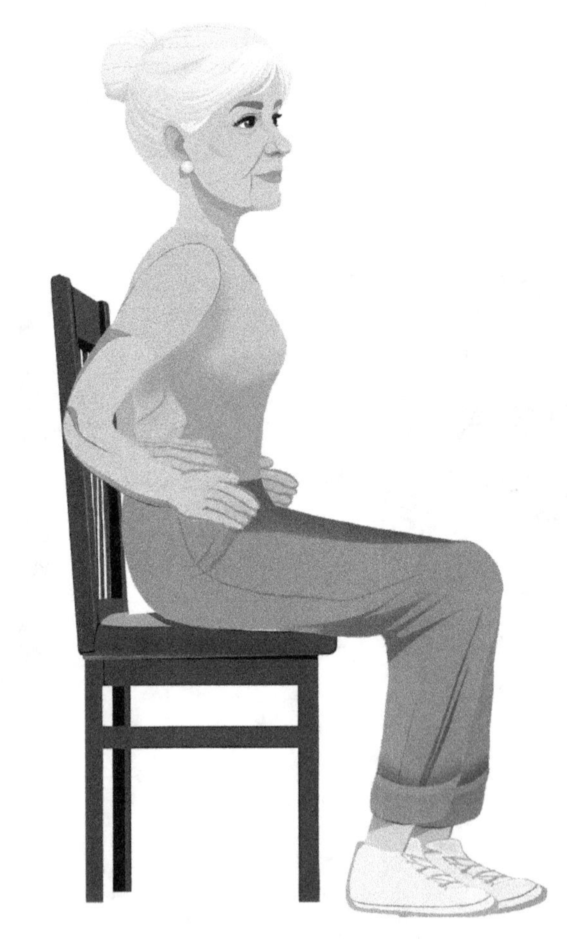

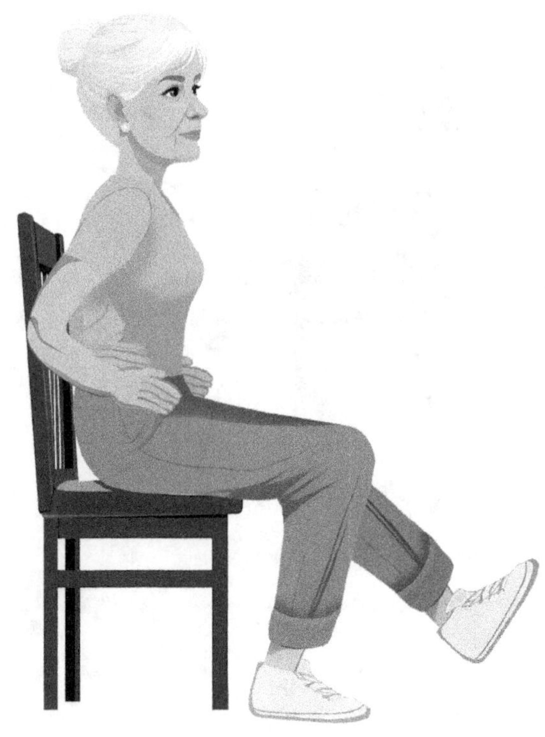

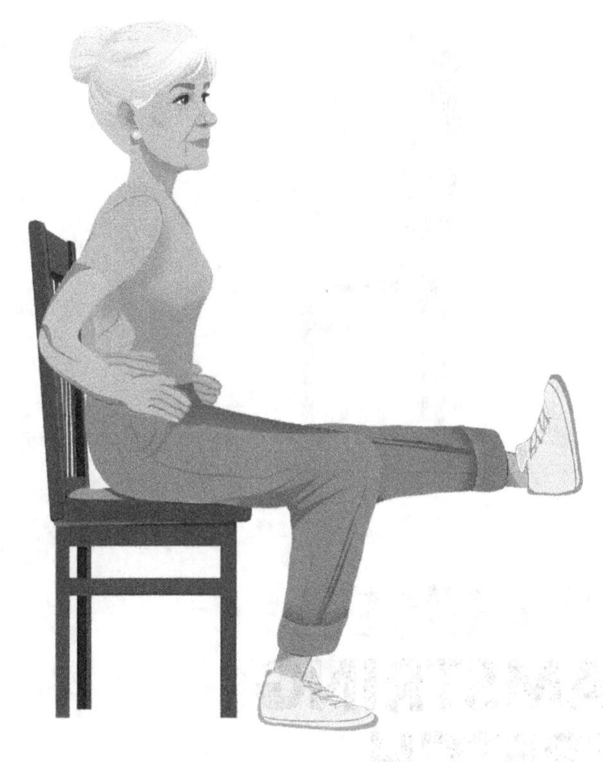

EXERCISE 3
TOE PUSH UPS

1. Sit upright on the edge of your chair with your hands resting on your thighs. Your feet should be together and heels on the floor.

2. Rise on your heels to perform toe raises. Feel the stretch in your calf muscles.

3. Lower your heels back to the floor.

4. Do ten repetitions, holding the last one for a count of five in the top position.

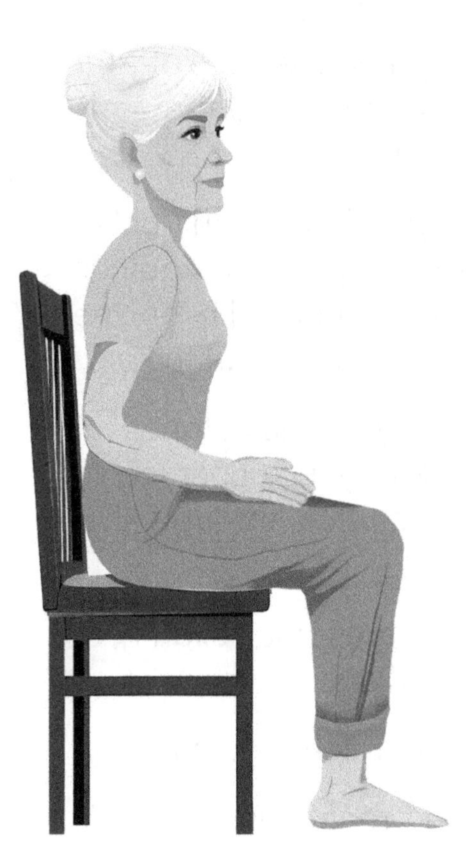

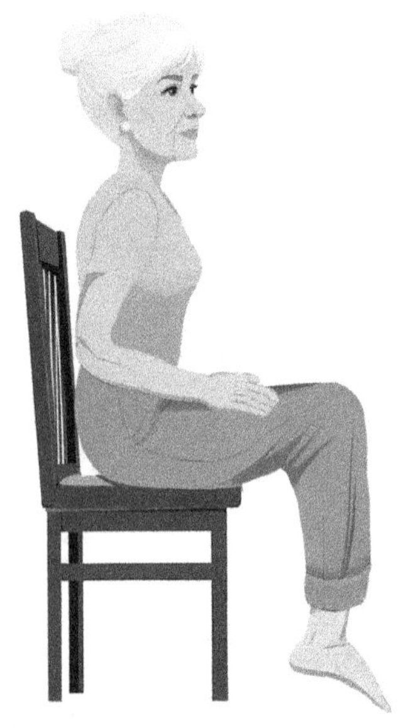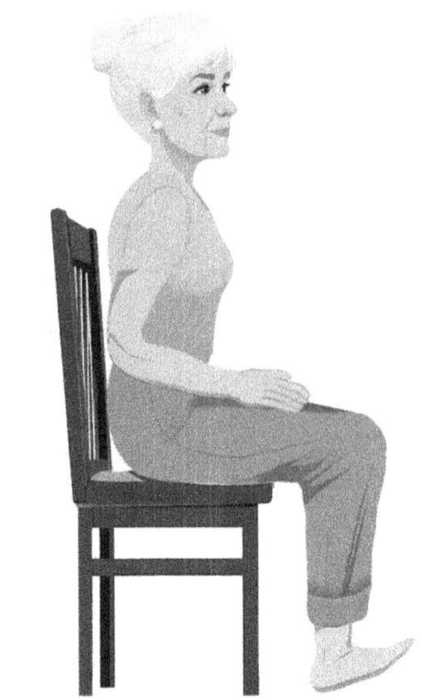

EXERCISE 4
HAMSTRING STRETCH

1. Sit upright on the edge of your chair and hold onto the arms of the chair.

2. Extend your legs out in front of you with your heels together. Your heels should be on the floor with your toes in the air,

3. Contract your hamstrings at the back of your upper leg to feel the stretch through that area.

4. Pull your toes back slightly to increase the stretch.

5. Flatten your feet to the floor.

6. Do ten repetitions of this stretch.

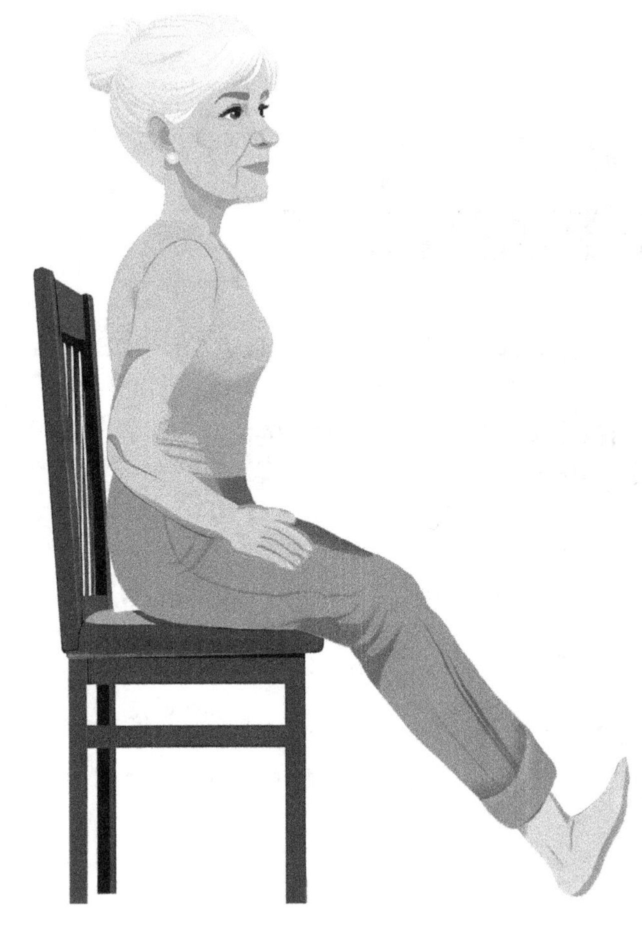

EXERCISE 5
ANKLE ROLL

1. Sit upright on the edge of the chair with your shoulder blades pulled back and hands on your thighs.

2. Place both hands under your right thigh and pull it up so the foot is about a foot off the ground.

3. Roll your raised foot five times to the left to maintain an upright torso.

4. Roll your foot five times to the right.

5. Repeat on the left leg.

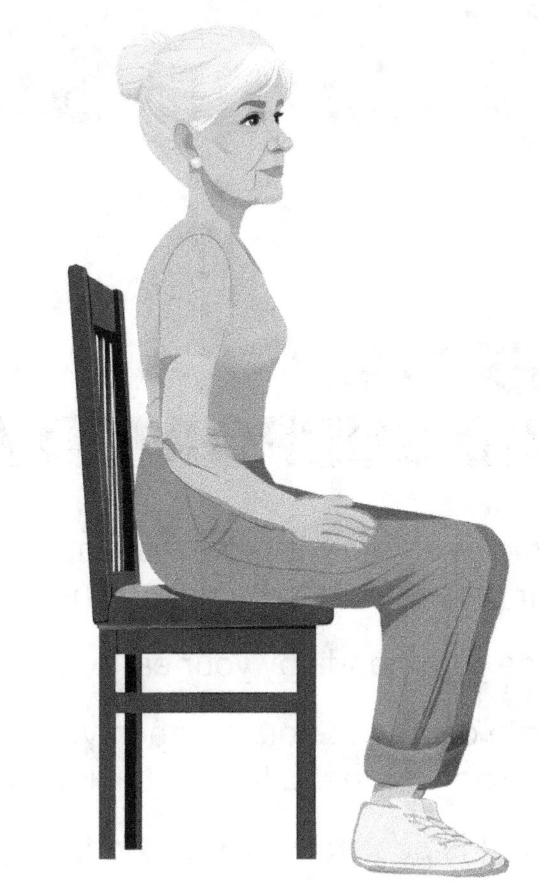

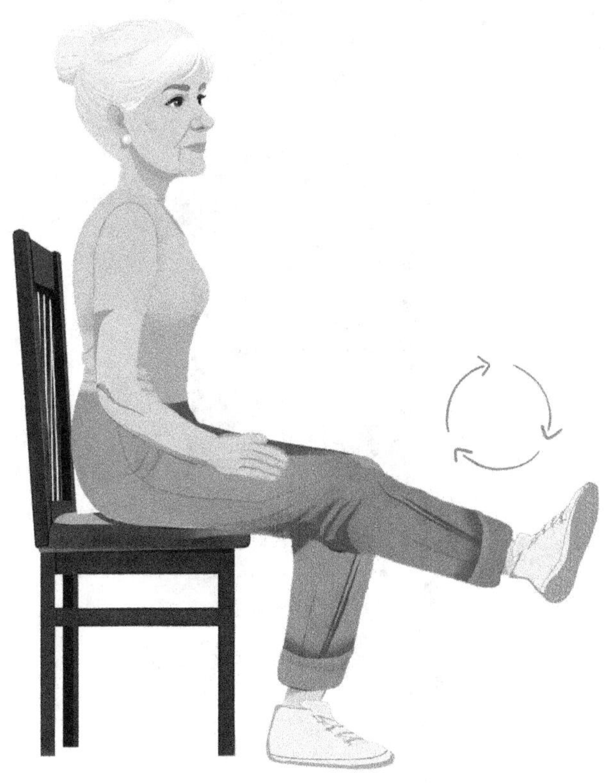

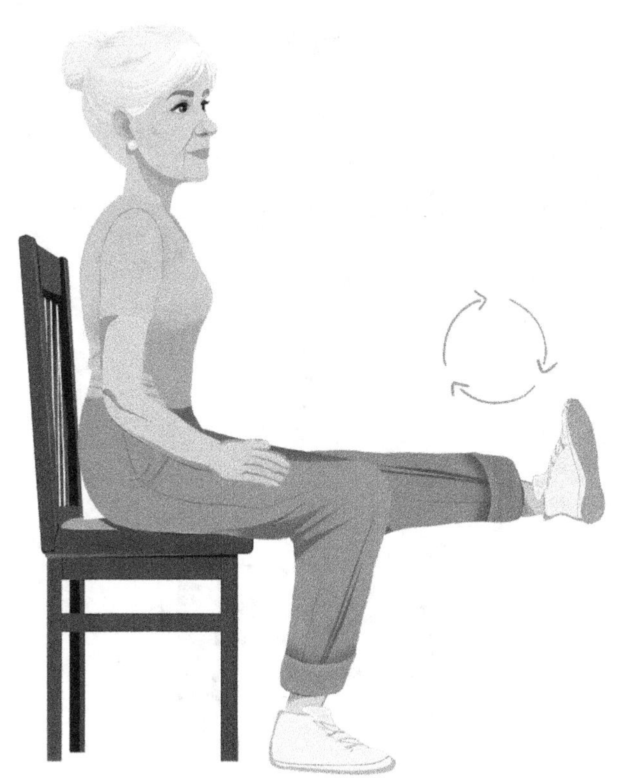

Upper Body Awareness

EXERCISE 1
HEAD SUPPORTED ARCH

1. Begin by sitting with your feet flat on the floor and your left foot in front. Sit tall, engaging your core and keeping your spine straight.

2. Place your hands by your ears.

3. Inhale deeply as you lengthen your spine. As you exhale, gently arch your upper back, allowing your head to lean back and be supported by the top of the chair's backrest.

4. Hold this pose for thirty seconds.

5. Do this exercise five times.

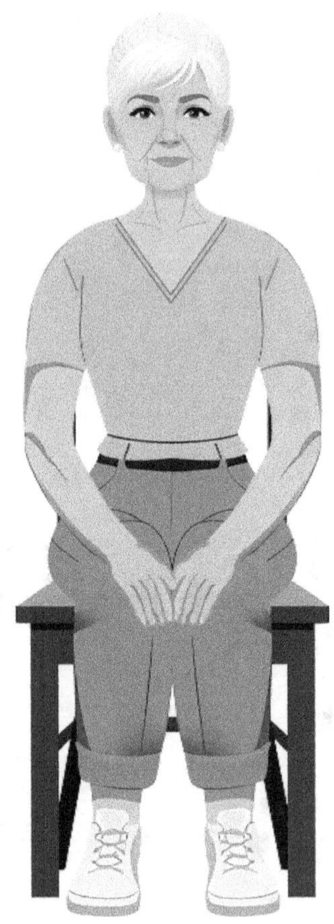

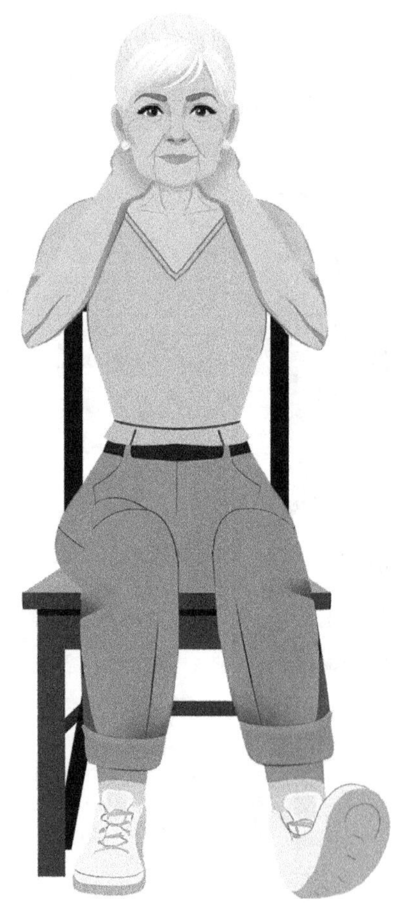

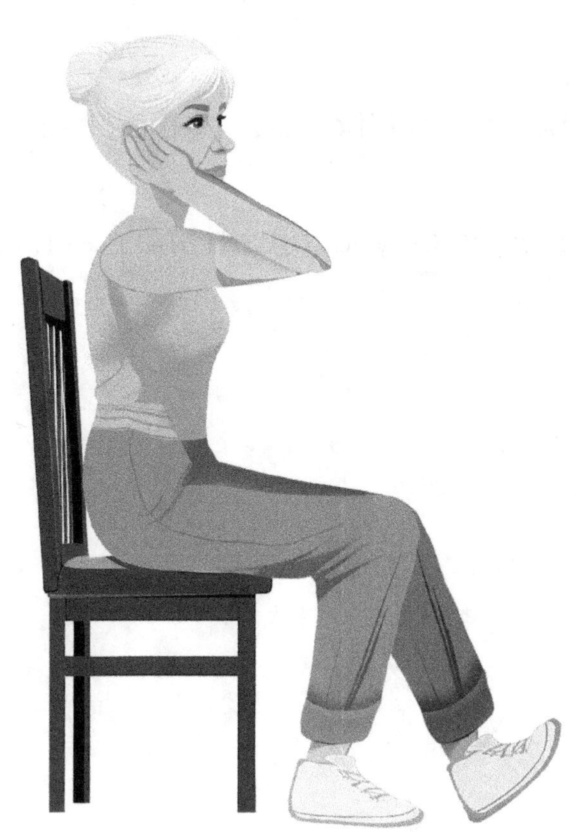

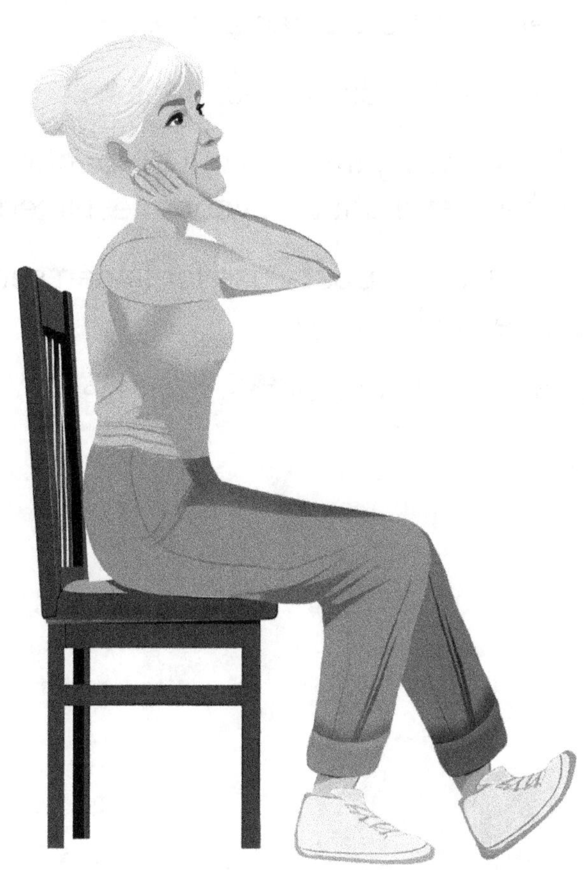

EXERCISE 2
CHAIR BOAT POSE

1. Sit with your back straight and your feet flat on the floor, hip-width apart. Now, slide forward to the edge of the chair.

2. Inhale as you lift your feet, bringing your shins parallel to the floor. Your knees should be bent at a 90-degree angle.

3. Place your hands on your knees.

4. Shift your weight onto your sit bones, finding balance on the edge of the chair. Keep your back straight and your chest lifted.

5. Hold the Chair Boat Pose for fifteen seconds, focusing on your breath and maintaining a stable position.

6. Do five repetitions of this exercise.

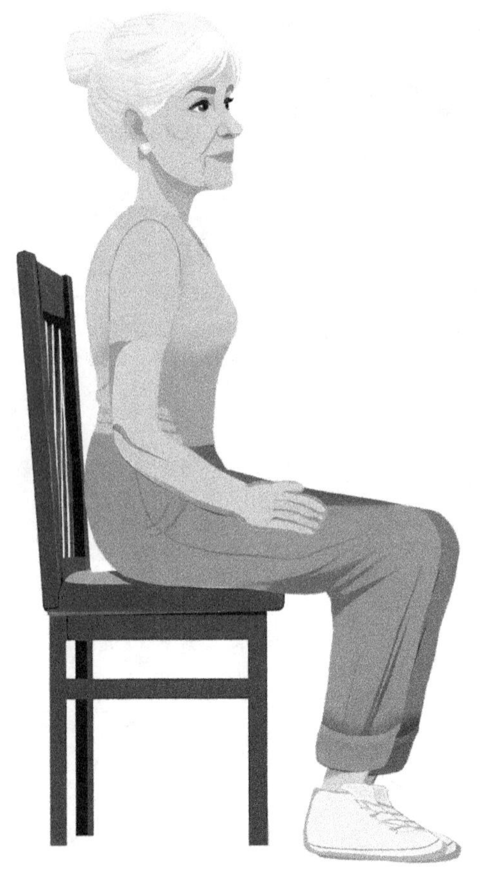

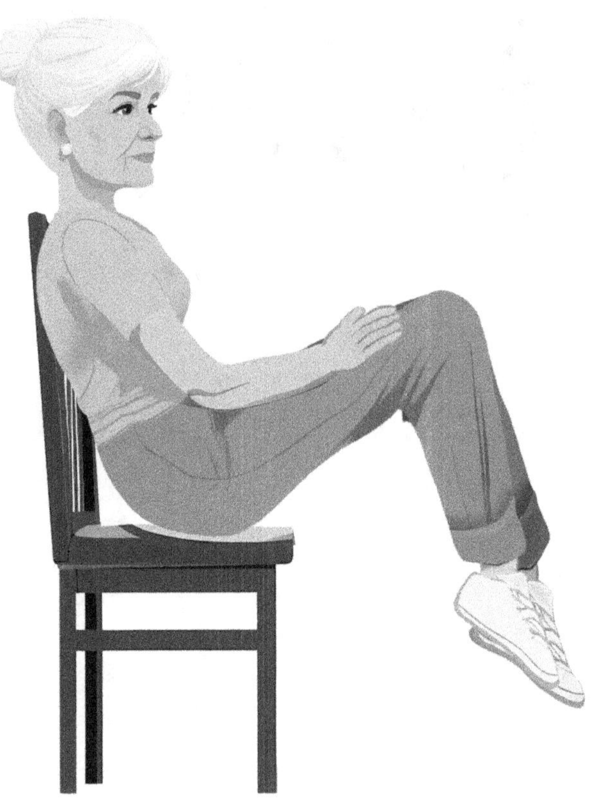

EXERCISE 3
CHAIR GODDESS POSE

1. Sit on the edge of the chair with your feet shoulder-width apart.

2. Slide your feet outward, opening your knees to the sides. Aim to bring your thighs parallel to the floor, forming a wide "V" shape with your legs.

3. Turn your toes slightly outward to accommodate the opening of the knees. Ensure your feet remain flat on the floor.

4. Bring your arms up to the "hands up" position. Push your shoulder blades down and extend your chest out in this position.

5. Hold the chair goddess pose for twenty seconds.

6. Do five reps of this exercise.

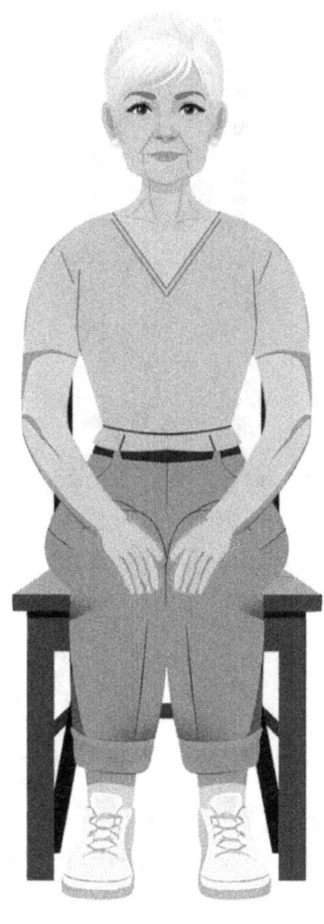
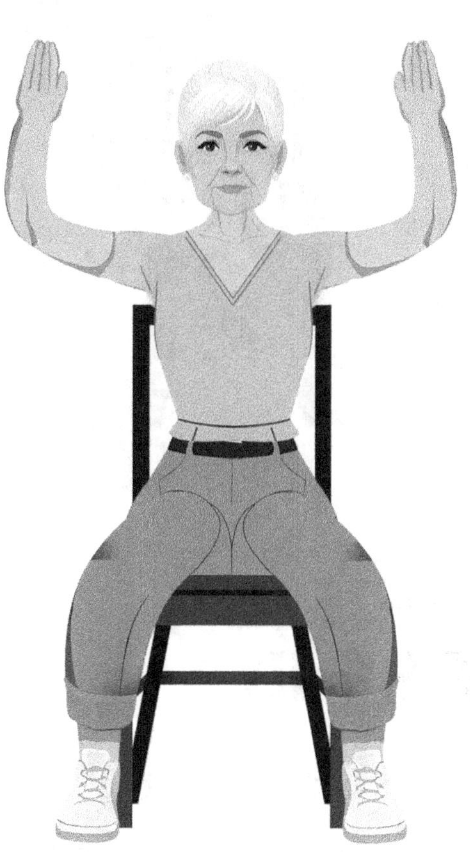

EXERCISE 4
CHAIR ARM CIRCLES

1. Sit up straight with your feet flat on the floor. Extend your arms straight out to the sides, parallel to the floor.

2. Begin making small circular motions with your arms, like you're drawing circles with your hands.

3. You can use an open-handed palm or your fists.

4. Continue the circular motions for ten seconds. Now, go in the other direction for ten seconds.

5. Do five repetitions of this exercise.

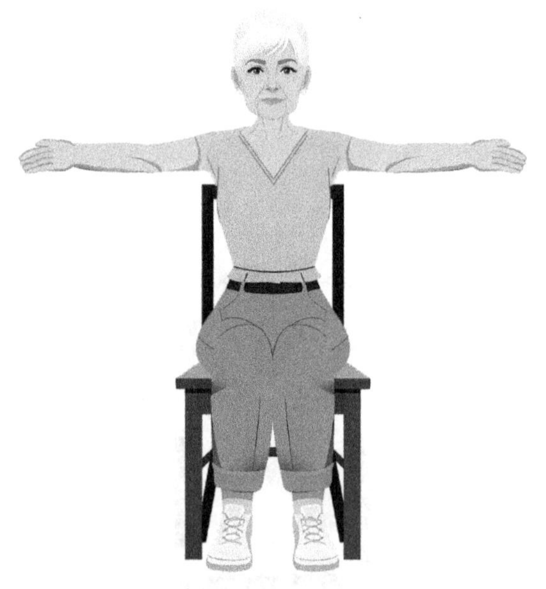 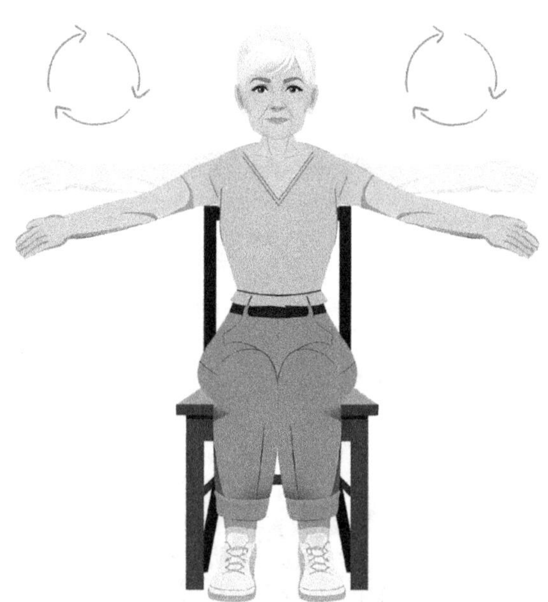

EXERCISE 5
SIDE BEND

1. Sit upright with your feet flat on the floor and your hands raised high in the air.

2. Take a few breaths and lengthen your spine. As you do, lean to the right with your hands leading.

3. Now return to the center and turn to the other side.

4. Perform ten reps on each side.

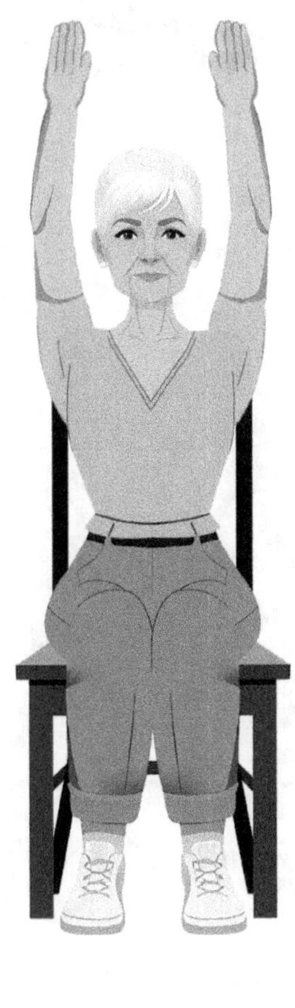

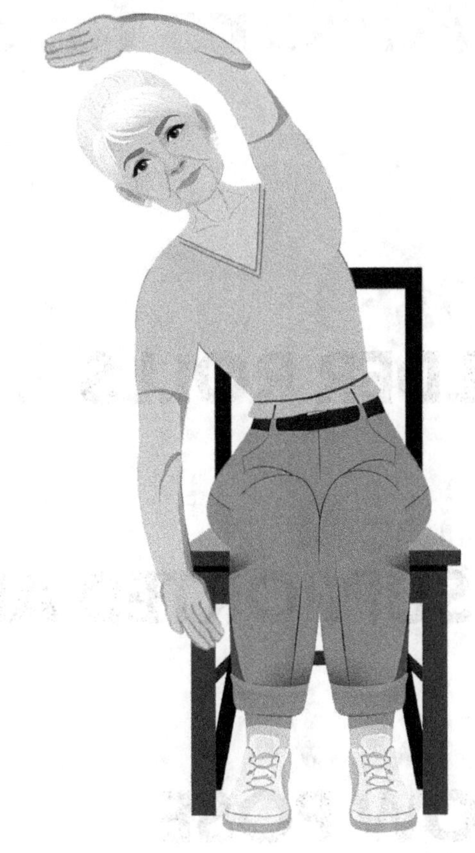

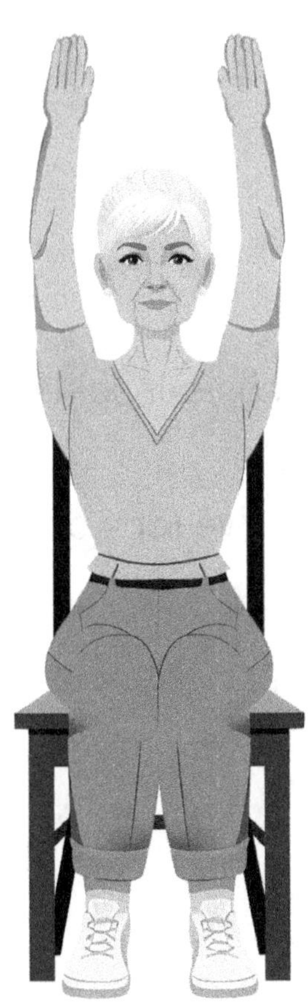

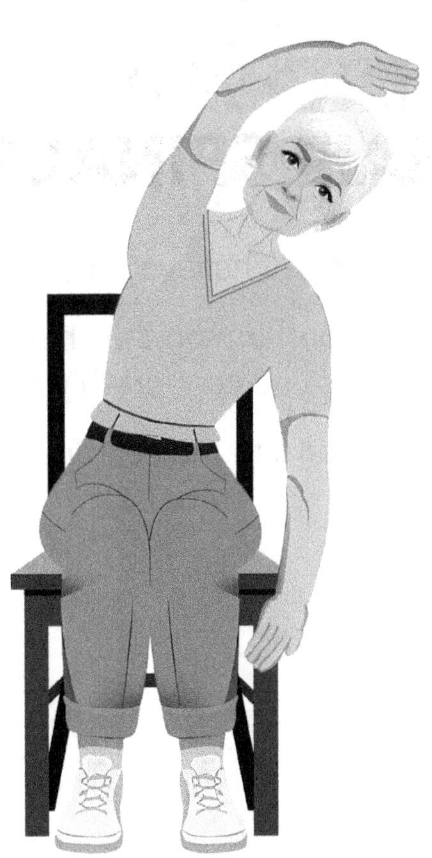

DAY 05 Posture Improvement

EXERCISE 1
SHOULDER ROLLS

EXERCISE 2
HEAD SUPPORTED ARCH

EXERCISE 3
CAT COW POSE

EXERCISE 4
CHAIR SPINAL TWIST

1. Sit on your chair, your back straight and chest up.

2. Place your arm on the chair's backrest and, as you lengthen your spine, turn backward as far as you comfortably can.

3. Now return to the center and turn to the other side. Do twelve reps on each side.

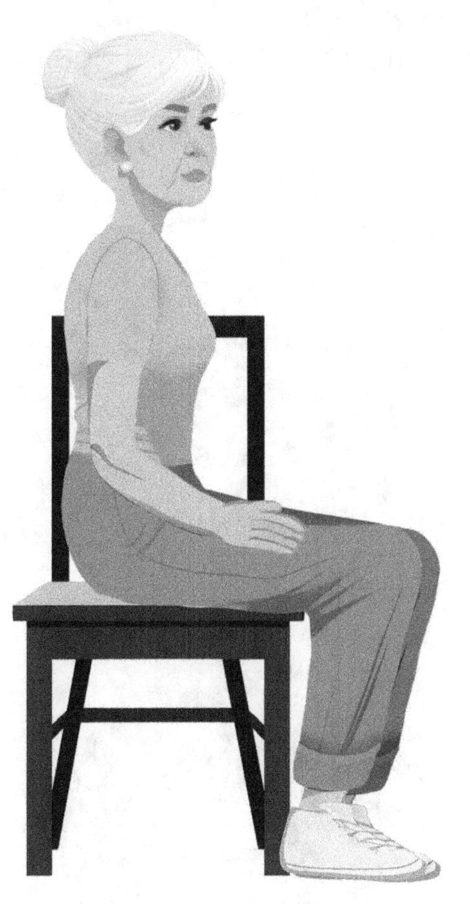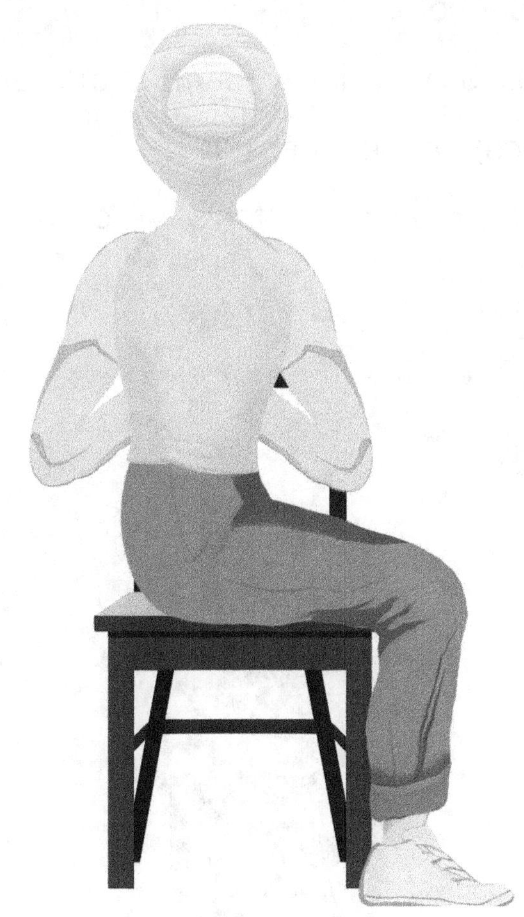

EXERCISE 5
CHAIR GODDESS TWIST

1. Sit on the edge of the chair with your feet shoulder-width apart.

2. Slide your feet outward, opening your knees to the sides. Aim to bring your thighs parallel to the floor, forming a wide "V" shape with your legs.

3. Turn your toes slightly outward to accommodate the opening of the knees. Ensure your feet remain flat on the floor.

4. Bring your arms up to the "hands up" position. Push your shoulder blades down and extend your chest out in this position.

5. Engage your core by drawing your navel toward your spine.

6. Exhale as you twist your upper body to the right, bringing your left hand up and overhead.

7. Turn your head to look up toward your extended hand.

8. Hold this position for fifteen seconds, breathing deeply and maintaining engagement

in your core.

9. Inhale as you slowly return to the center, bringing your arms overhead again.

10. Repeat on the other side.

11. Do five repetitions of this exercise.

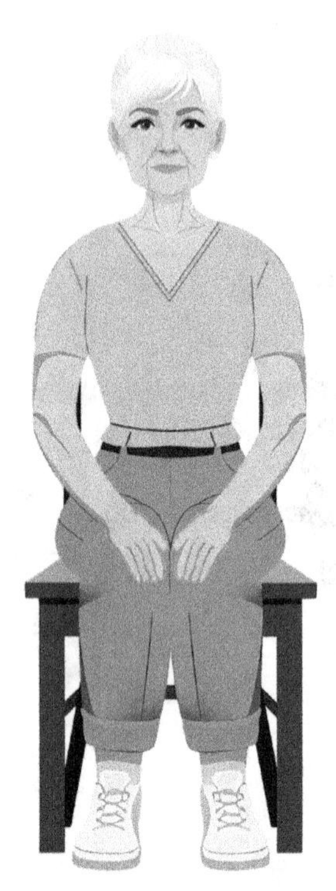

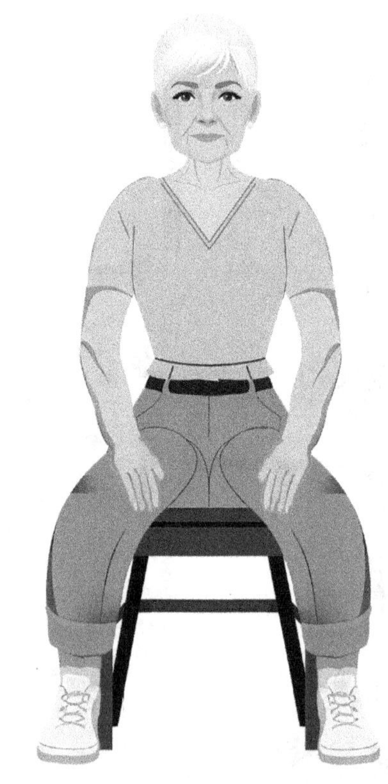

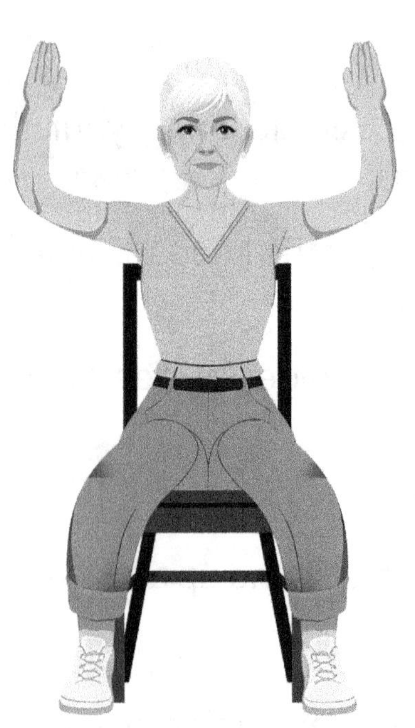

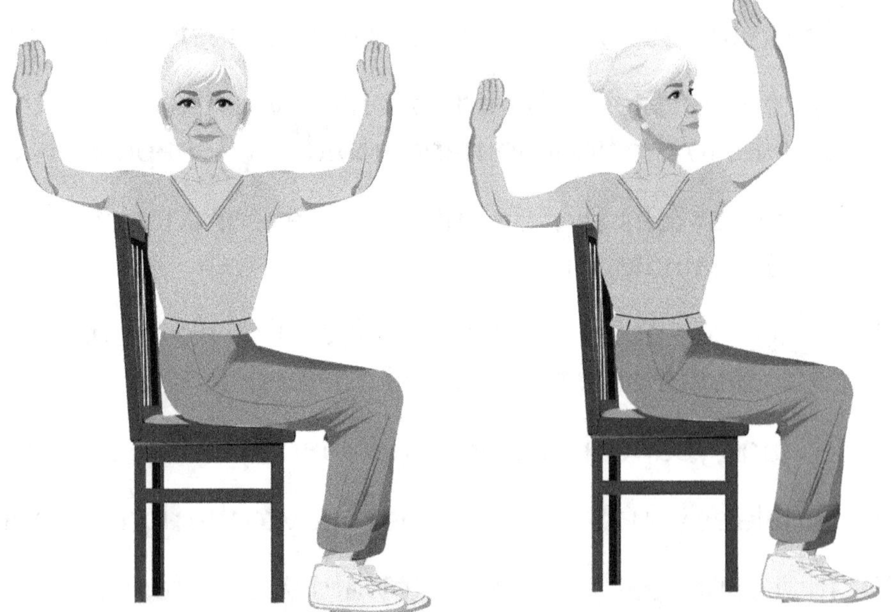

DAY Relaxation/
06 Stress Reduction Poses

EXERCISE 1
CAMEL POSE

1. Get down on your knees with your back to the chair. Sit on your heels in an upright position.

2. Extend your arms behind you to touch the sides of the chair with your hands facing downward.

3. Breathe deeply as you arch back to stretch through your spine.

4. Hold for 30 seconds.

5. Perform 5 repetitions of this exercise.

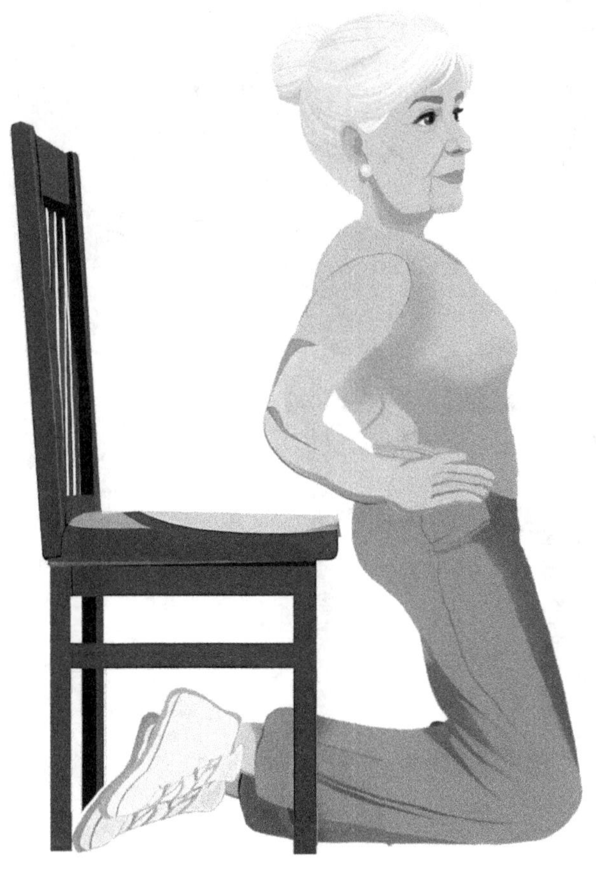
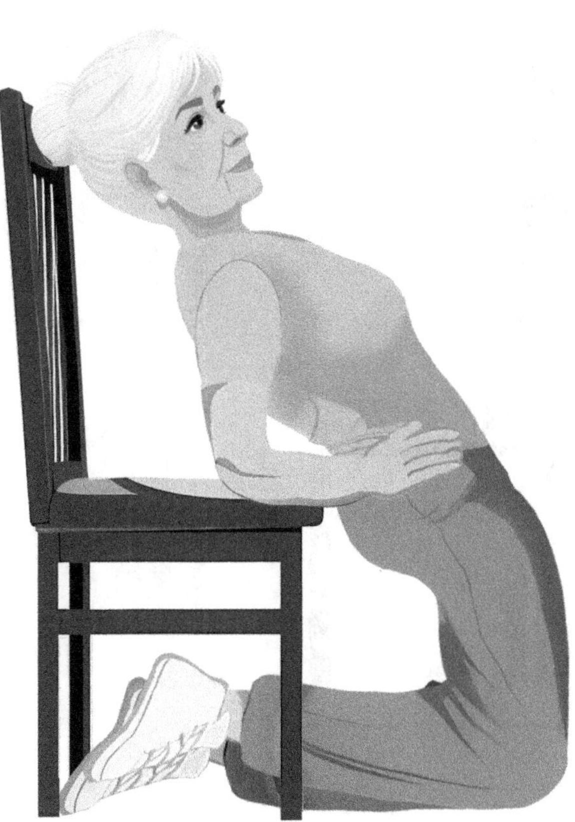

EXERCISE 2
CHAIR DOWNWARD DOG

1. Stand in front of your chair with your feet shoulder-width apart.

2. Bend at the hips to bend down and take hold of the sides of the chair. Your arms should be fully extended in this position, and your back should be straight.

3. Without bending your arms, lift your hips into the air. Shuffle forward slightly until your body forms an inverted 'V' shape.

4. Drop your head and extend your spine in this position. Hold for 15 seconds.

5. Perform 5 repetitions of this exercise.

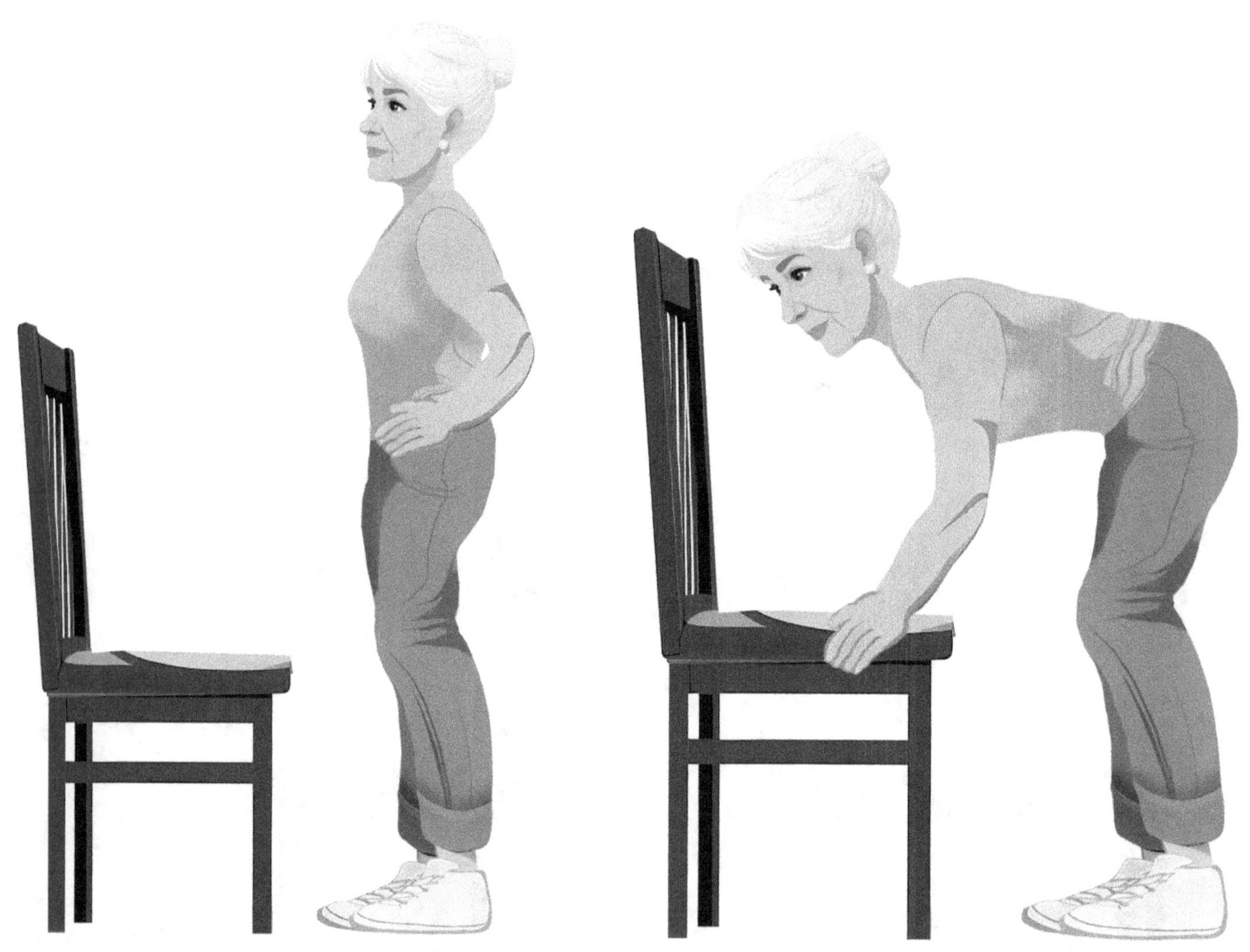

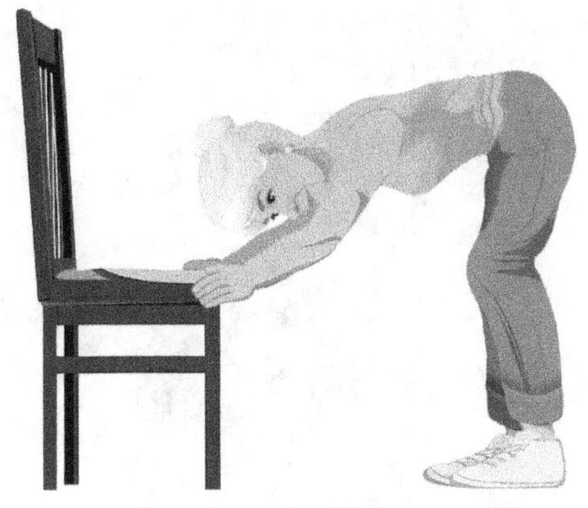 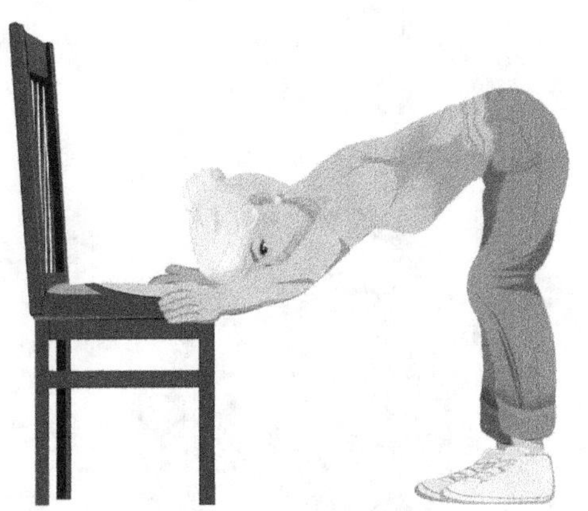

EXERCISE 3
SEATED EXTENDED SIDE ANGLE POSE

1. Sit with your back straight and your feet flat on the floor, hip-width apart. Slide forward to the edge of the chair.

2. Extend your right leg out to the side, keeping it straight. Your toes should be pointing forward or slightly angled upwards.

3. Keep your left foot firmly planted on the floor, ensuring it aligns with your hip.

4. Inhale deeply as you raise your right arm overhead, reaching towards the ceiling. Rest your right forearm on your right thigh. Your right side should feel a stretch from your fingertips down to your hip.

5. Hold the seated extended side angle pose for fifteen seconds.

6. Repeat on the other side.

7. Do this exercise five times.

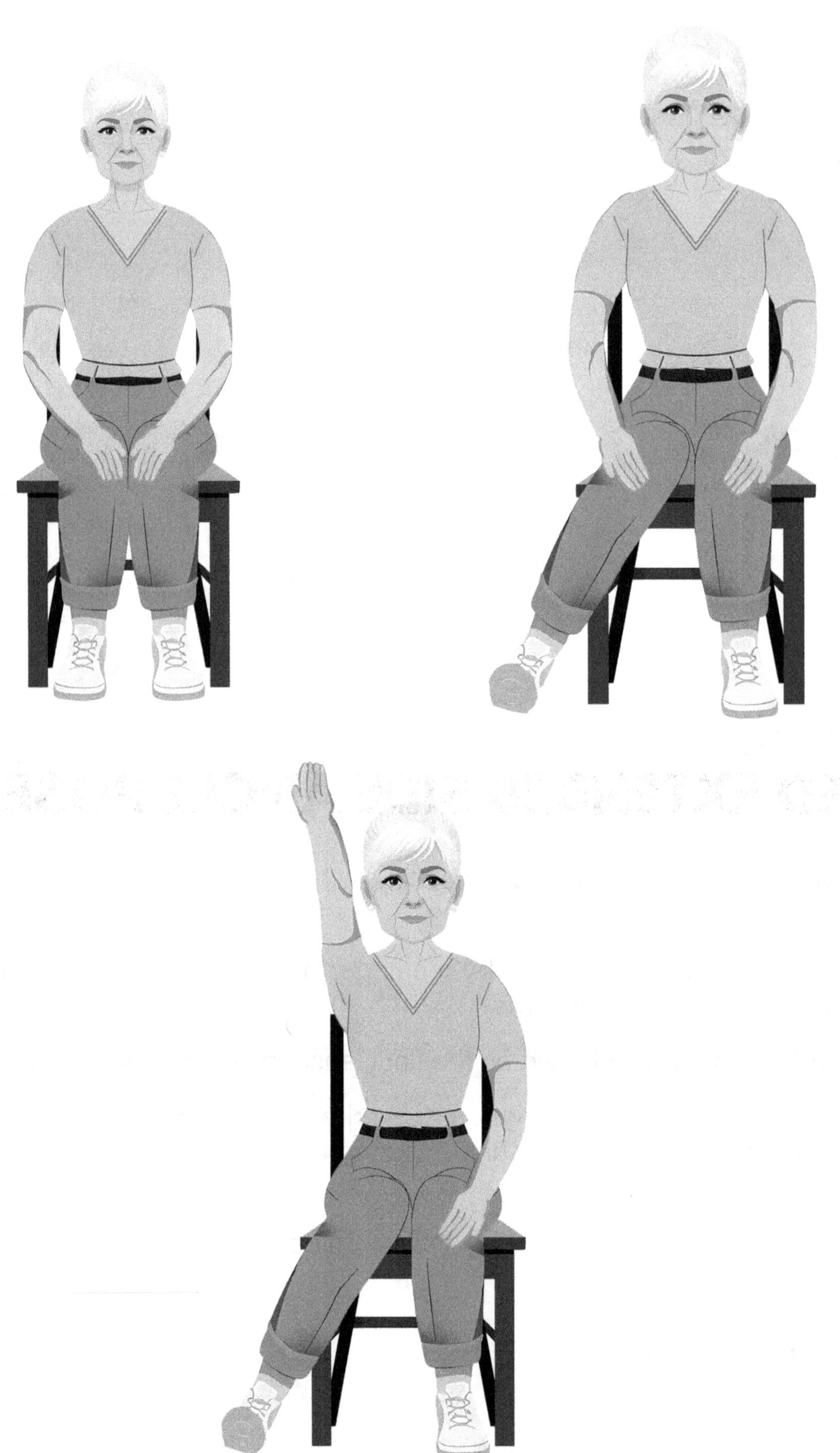

EXERCISE 4
ELBOW REACH

1. Sit comfortably on your chair with your feet flat on the floor, hip-width apart. Ensure that your back is straight and your shoulders are relaxed.

2. Extend your arms overhead, then bend your elbows so that your forearms are parallel to the floor. Place your hands over the opposite elbow.

3. Expand your chest and reach up into the stretch.

4. Hold the pose for thirty seconds, feeling a comfortable stretch.

5. Do 5 repetitions of this exercise.

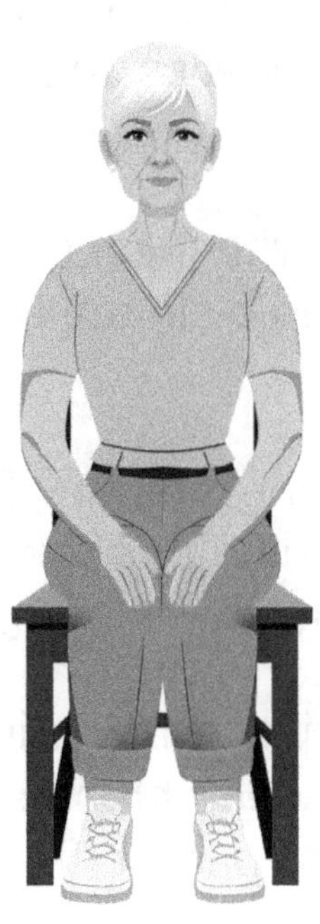
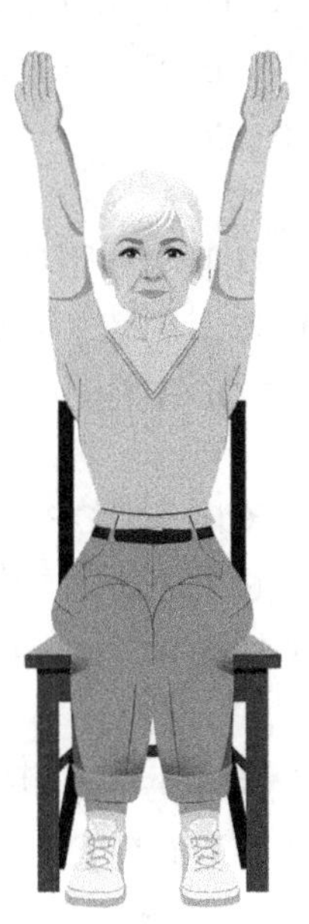
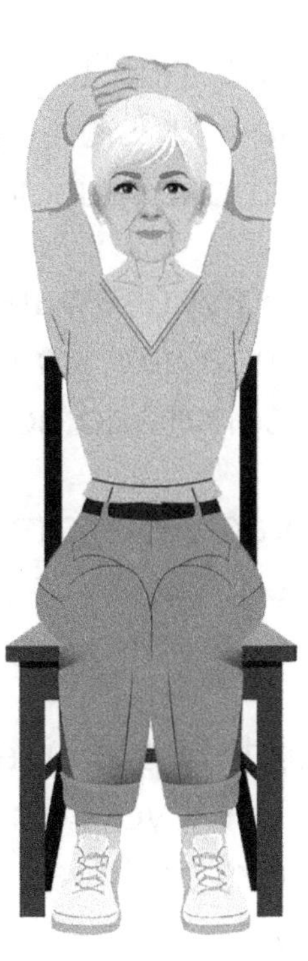

EXERCISE 5
HEAD-SUPPORTED ARCH

Do 3 repetitions of this exercise.

DAY 07 Mindful Relaxation

Today, you will give your body a break from chair yoga exercises. Instead, you will lie on the floor (or your bed) and practice mindful meditation. You will want to do this at a time and place that allows for quiet peacefulness.

Once you've located your area, lie on your back with your arms at your sides, palms down, and close your eyes gently. Take a deep breath through your nose, feeling your lungs expand fully, and then exhale slowly through your mouth, releasing any tension you may be holding onto. Allow your body to sink into the floor or bed beneath you.

As you continue to breathe deeply and rhythmically, bring your attention to your body. Notice any tension or discomfort; with each exhale, consciously release that tension, allowing those muscles to soften and relax.

Now, bring your awareness to your thoughts. Rather than engaging with them or trying to push them away, simply observe them as if they were clouds passing by in the sky. Allow them to come and go without judgment or attachment.

As you practice this mindful meditation, remember to stay present in the moment, focusing on the sensations of your breath and the feeling of relaxation spreading throughout your body. If your mind starts to wander, gently guide your attention back to your breath.

Continue this practice for as long as it feels comfortable, whether just a few minutes or longer. When you're ready to conclude your meditation, take a few deep breaths, wiggle your fingers and toes, and slowly open your eyes, bringing awareness back to the present moment.

Take a moment to notice how you feel after this period of mindful relaxation. Allow yourself to carry this sense of calm and ease as you go about the rest of your day, including your daily chair yoga sessions.

STRENGTH
LOWER BODY & CORE

This week, your focus is on building strength through your body's base. By strengthening your quadriceps, hamstrings, glutes, calves, and core, you will establish a foundation of support to keep your body secure and stable on any surface.

You will be performing two rounds of each four-exercise circuit. Move through each circuit at a slightly challenging pace but not overwhelming for you. Then, rest for 2-3 minutes before repeating the circuit.

DAY 08 Lower Body Strength

EXERCISE 1
LEG EXTENSION

Do 12 repetitions of this exercise.

EXERCISE 2
LEG DRAG

1. Sit upright on the edge of your chair and hold the sides of the chair for support.

2. Extend your right foot before you, keeping your entire foot on the ground.

3. Drag your right leg back toward the seat. You will feel your hamstring working as you do this.

4. Repeat for 12 repetitions.

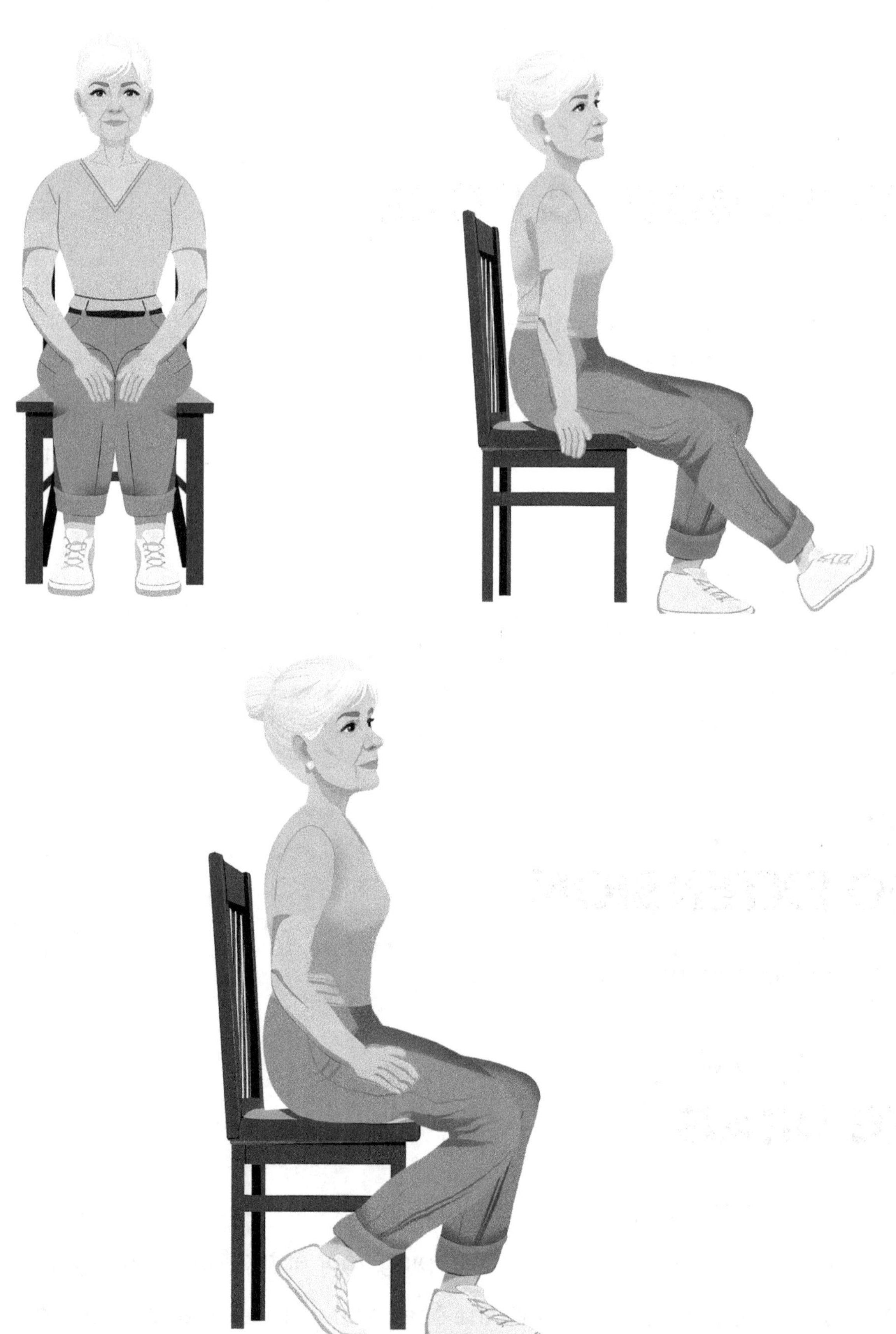

EXERCISE 3
LATERAL LEG LIFT

1. Sit upright on the edge of your chair and hold the sides for support. Your legs should be bent at right angles, and your feet should be firmly planted on the floor.

2. Lift your right knee directly up and to the right, rotating the hip in that direction.

3. Tap the floor with your right foot and then lift the knee to return to the start position.

4. Do 12 repetitions and then repeat on the left side.

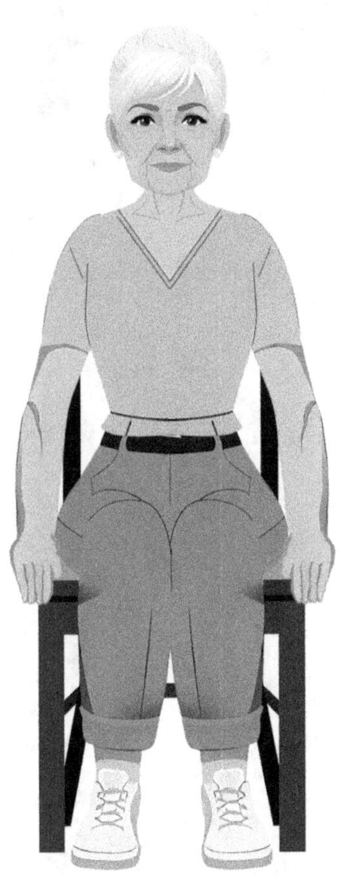
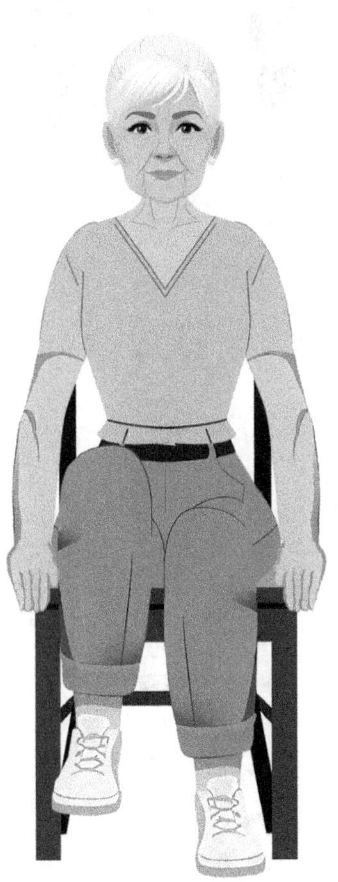

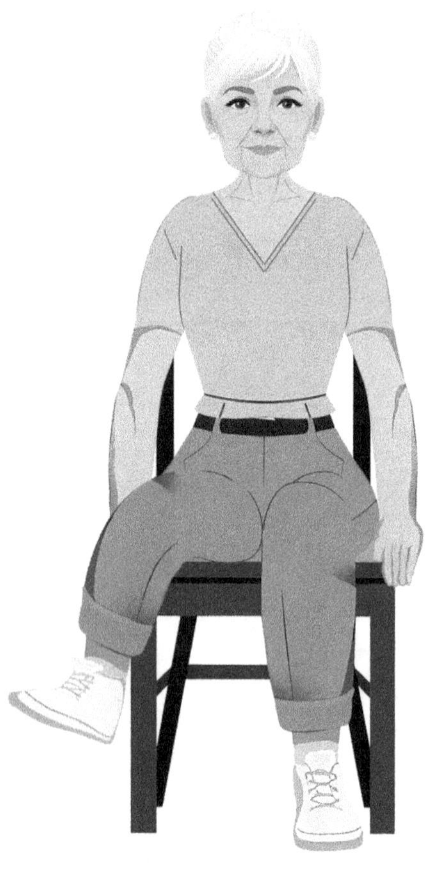
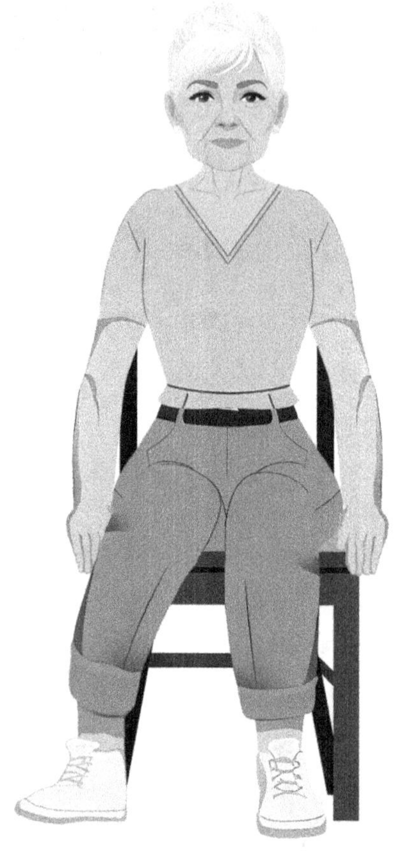
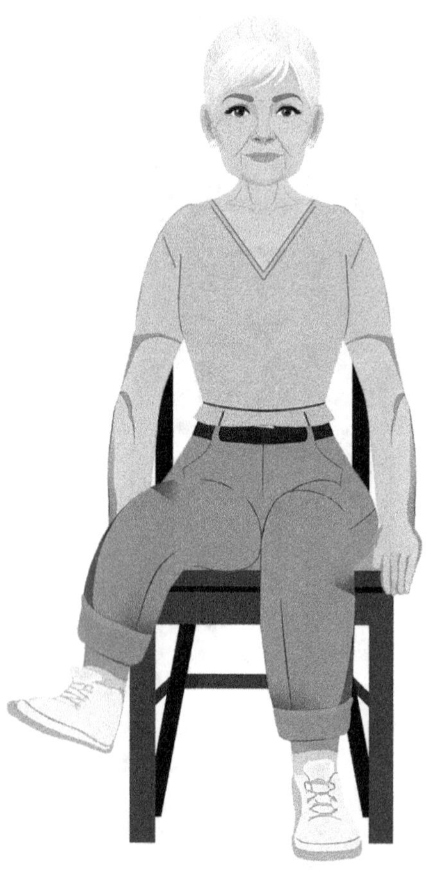
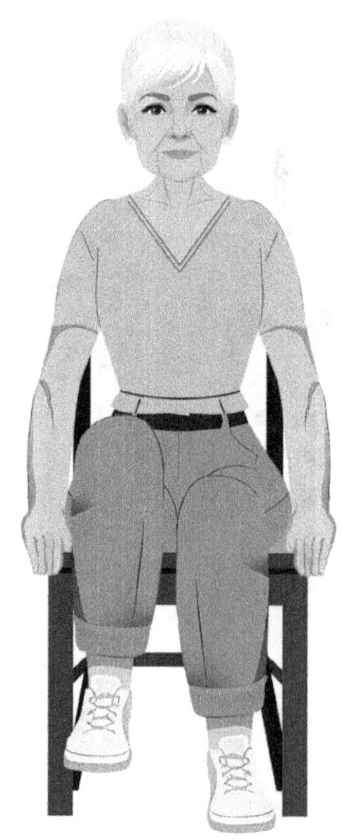

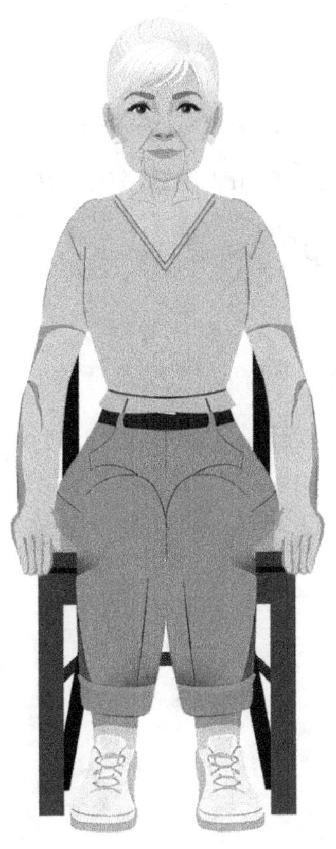 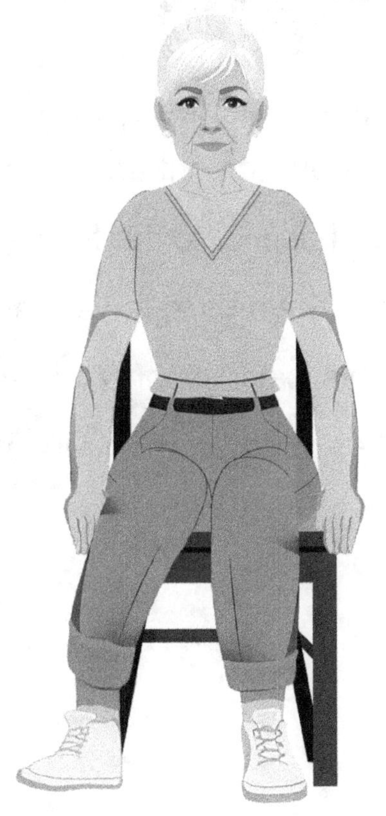

EXERCISE 4
SIT & STAND

1. Sit upright on the edge of your chair with your hands clasped in front of you. Your legs should be bent at right angles, and your feet should be firmly planted on the floor.

2. Press your heels onto the floor as you rise to a standing position.

3. Hinge from the hips to lower back down into the chair.

4. Perform this exercise for 5 repetitions.

5. Rest for 2-3 minutes, then repeat these four exercises.

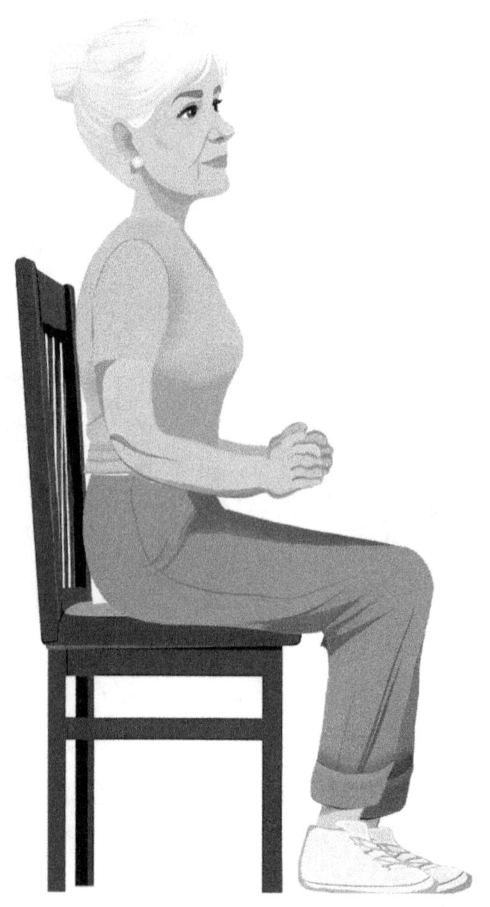
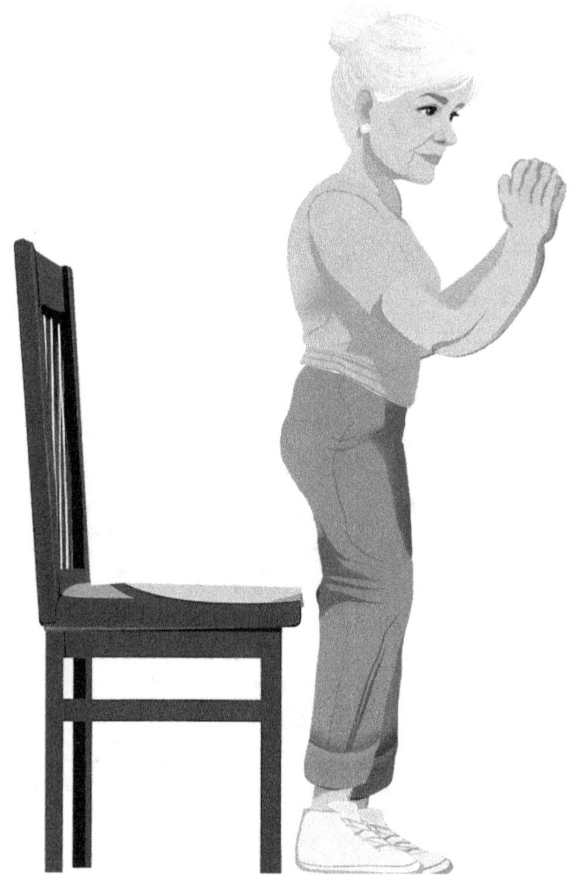

DAY 09 Core Strength

EXERCISE 1
CHAIR SPINAL TWIST

Do 12 repetitions of this exercise.

EXERCISE 2
CHAIR GODDESS TWIST

Do 12 repetitions of this exercise.

EXERCISE 3
CHAIR BOAT POSE

Do 12 repetitions of this exercise.

EXERCISE 4
MOUNTAIN CLIMBER

Do 12 repetitions of this exercise.

1. Position yourself facing the chair and place your hands on the seat shoulder-width apart.

2. Step back to create a plank position, with your body forming a straight line from head to heels. Keep your wrists directly under your shoulders and your feet hip-width apart.

3. Lean into the chair for added support, distributing your weight evenly between your hands.

4. Lift your right knee toward your chest, engage your core muscles, and kick the leg back. Alternate legs dynamically and controlled, simulating a running motion. Focus on bringing your knees as close to your chest as comfortably as possible.

5. Perform the mountain climber at a pace that challenges you but allows for proper form. Maintain a smooth, controlled rhythm to enhance the exercise's effectiveness.

6. Perform ten repetitions on each leg.

7. Rest for 2-3 minutes, then repeat these four exercises.

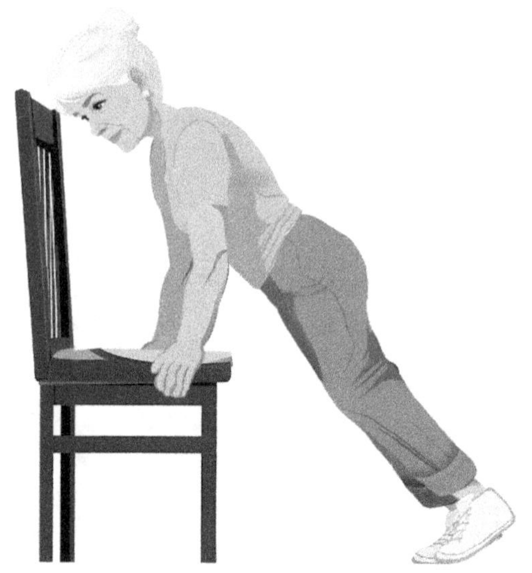
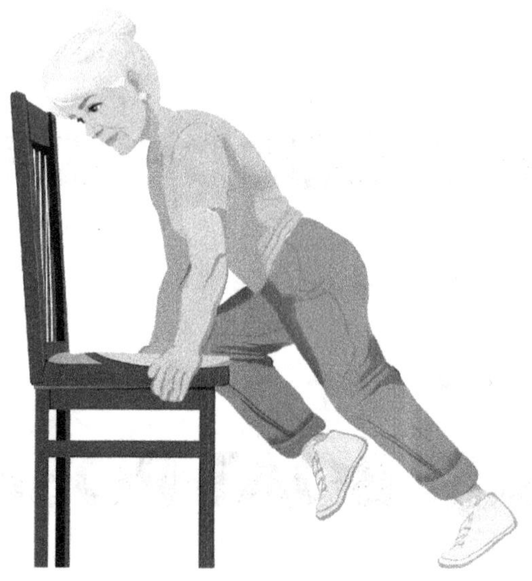
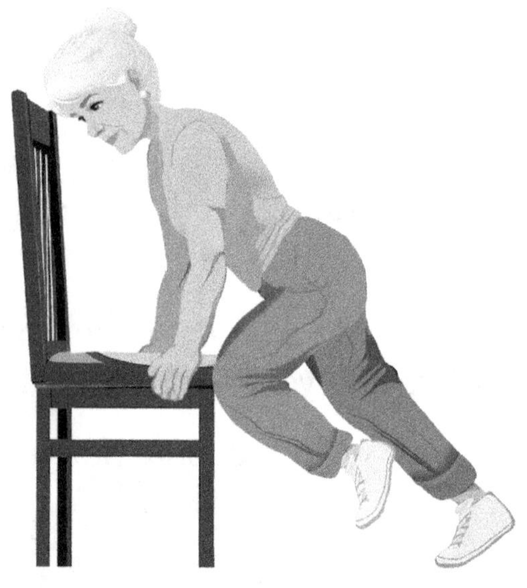
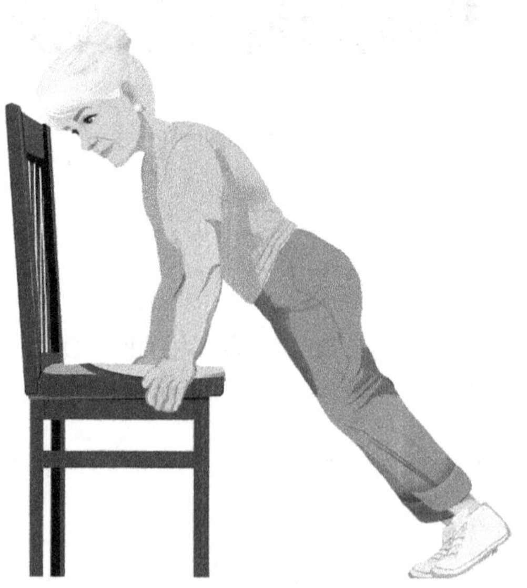

DAY 10 Lower Body/ Core Endurance

EXERCISE 1
LEG SHUFFLE

1. Sit on a chair with your back straight and your legs extended in front of you, hip-width apart. Grasp the sides of the chair for support.

2. Lift both feet slightly off the ground and shuffle them across each other in scissor fashion. Continue this side-to-side shuffling motion.

3. Perform the shuffling movement at a controlled and deliberate pace. Focus on maintaining balance and control throughout the exercise, avoiding any sudden or jerky movements.

4. Do fifteen repetitions of this exercise.

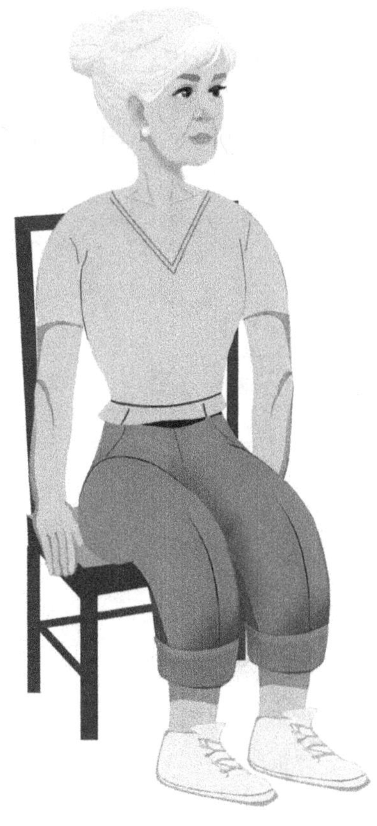

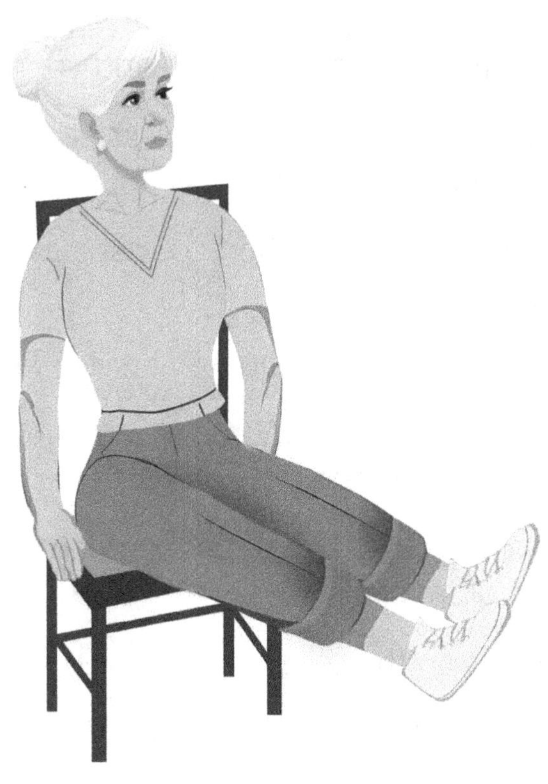

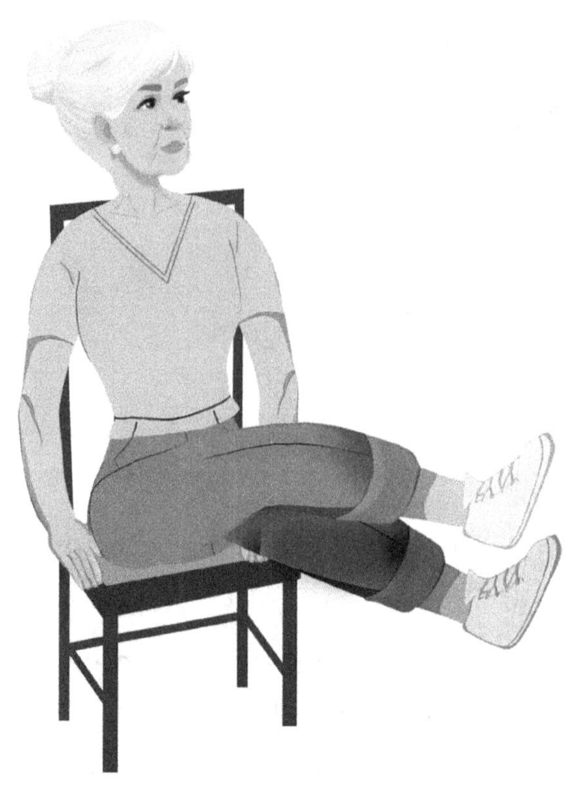

EXERCISE 2
CROSS LEG SIDE BEND

1. Sit with your back straight and your feet flat on the floor, hip-width apart.

2. Bring your right ankle to rest on your left knee. If this is uncomfortable, simply cross your legs at the ankles.

3. Inhale as you lengthen your spine, sitting up tall. Imagine your head reaching towards the ceiling.

4. Place your right hand on your left knee and raise your left arm.

5. Gently stretch your torso to the right by bringing your right arm over your head. Feel the stretch along the right side of your torso.

6. Hold the stretch for fifteen seconds, breathing deeply and maintaining a comfortable level of tension.

7. Repeat on the other side.

8. Do five reps on this exercise.

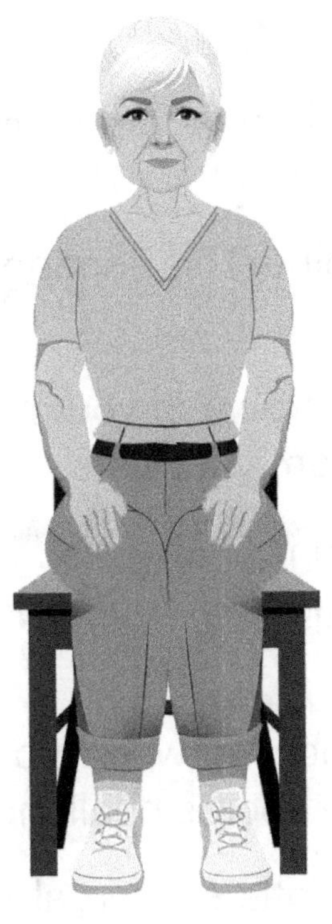

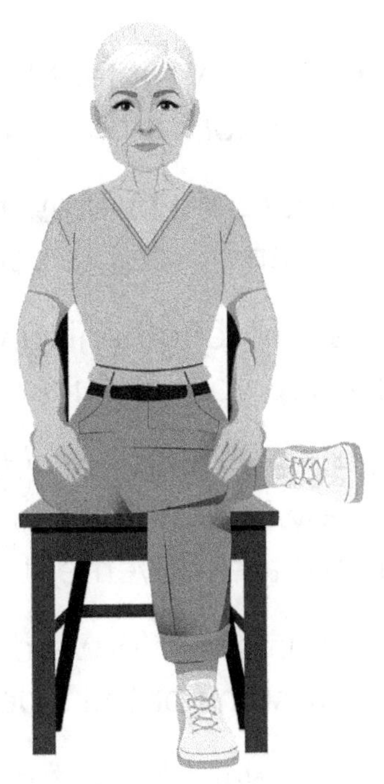

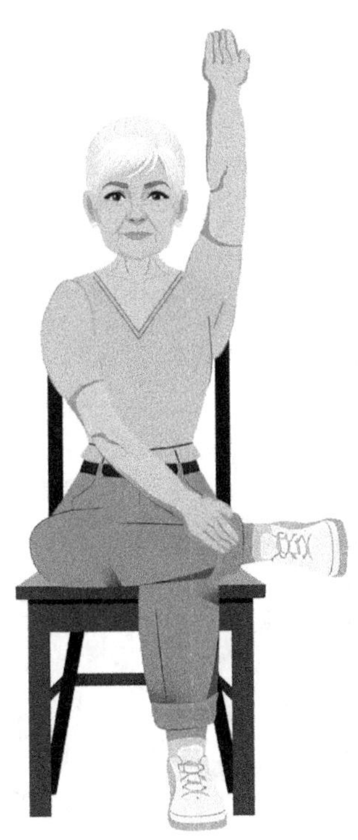

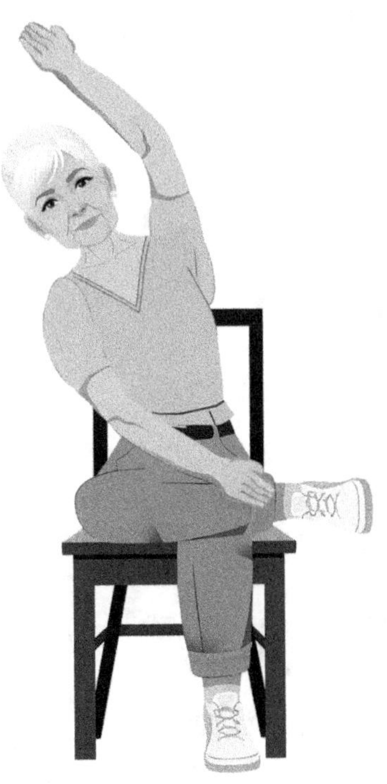

EXERCISE 3
FORWARD BEND

1. Sit upright with your feet flat on the floor. Sit toward the front edge of the chair to allow space for the forward bend.

2. Activate your core by drawing your navel toward your spine. This engagement supports movement and protects your lower back.

3. Inhale deeply, lengthening your spine and reaching the crown of your head toward the ceiling. Keep your shoulders relaxed and down, away from your ears.

4. As you exhale, hinge at your hips and lean forward from your waist. Lead with your chest, allowing your torso to descend toward your thighs. Keep your back straight throughout the movement.

5. Extend your arms forward toward the floor or the space between your feet. Aim to touch your shins or the sides of your feet if reaching the floor is challenging.

6. Hold the forward bend for fifteen seconds, feeling a gentle stretch along your spine, hamstrings, and hips. Focus on relaxing and breathing deeply during the stretch.

7. Inhale as you slowly return to an upright seated position, engaging your core to support the ascent.

8. Do five repetitions of this exercise.

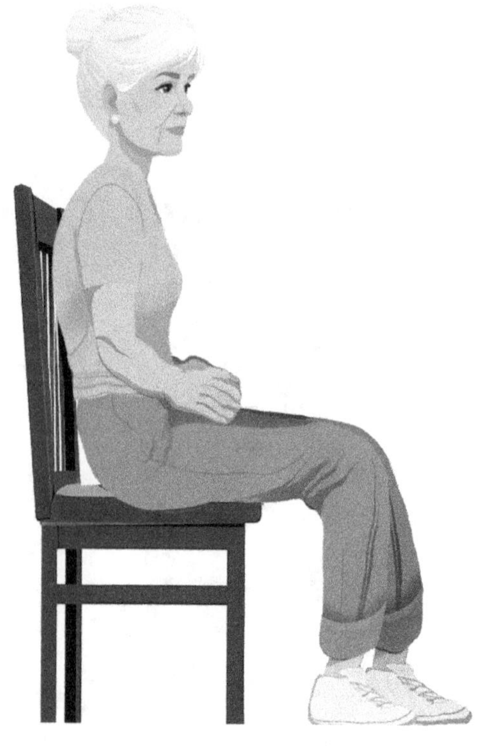
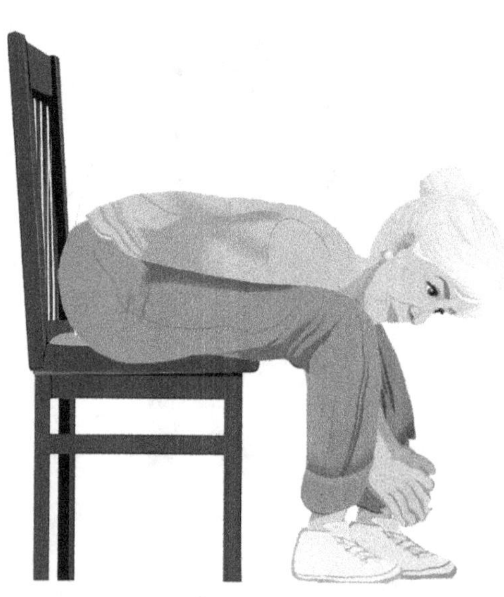

EXERCISE 4
MOUNTAIN CLIMBERS

Do 12 reps on each leg.

Rest for 2-3 minutes, then repeat these four exercises.

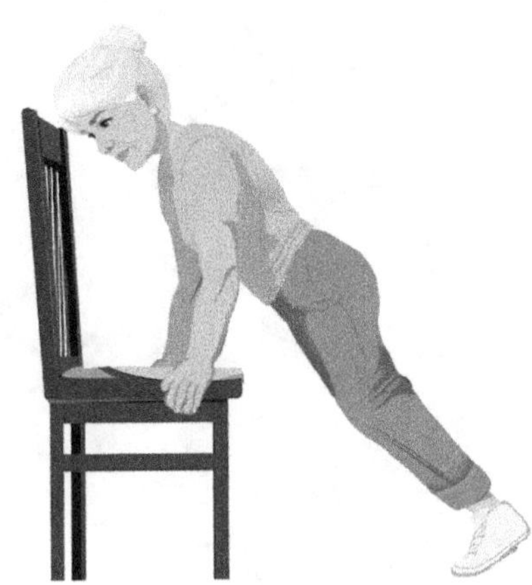
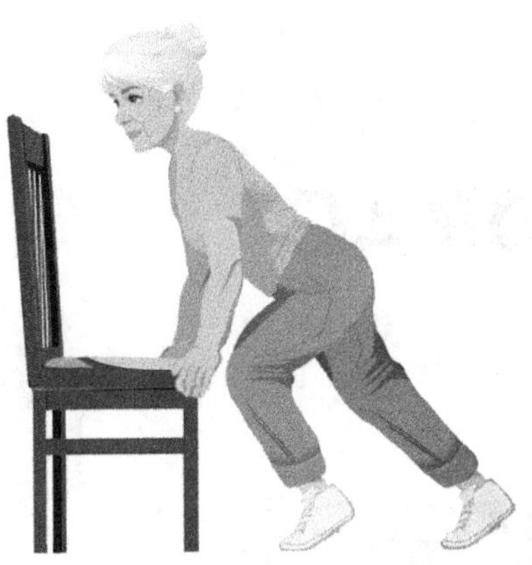
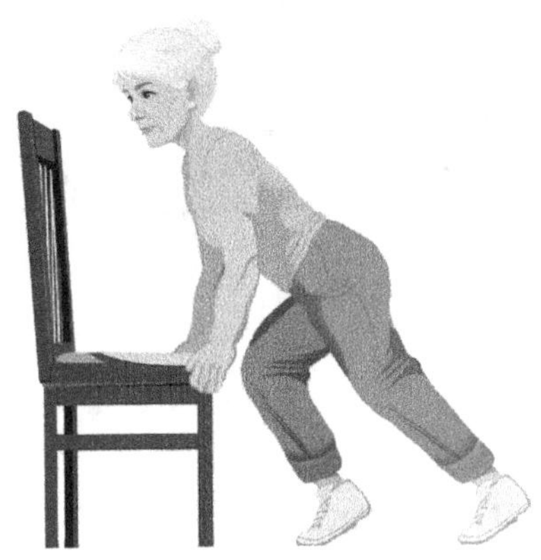

DAY 11 Lower Body Strength

EXERCISE 1
LEG EXTENSION

Do 12 repetitions of this exercise on each leg.

EXERCISE 2
LEG DRAG

Do 12 repetitions of this exercise on each leg.

EXERCISE 3
LATERAL LEG LIFT

Do 12 repetitions of this exercise on each leg.

EXERCISE 4
SIT & STAND

Do 5 repetitions of this exercise.

Rest for 2-3 minutes, then repeat these four exercises.

DAY 12 Core Strength

EXERCISE 1
CHAIR SPINAL TWIST

Do 12 repetitions of this exercise.

EXERCISE 2
CHAIR GODDESS TWIST

Do 12 repetitions of this exercise.

EXERCISE 3
CHAIR BOAT POSE

Do 12 repetitions of this exercise.

EXERCISE 4
MOUNTAIN CLIMBER

Do 12 repetitions of this exercise.

Rest for 2-3 minutes, then repeat these four exercises.

DAY 13
Isometric Strength

EXERCISE 1
CHAIR SQUAT HOLD

1. Sit upright on the edge of your chair with your hands clasped in front of you. Your legs should be bent at right angles, and your feet should be firmly planted on the floor.

2. Press your heels onto the floor as you rise to a standing position.

3. Hinge from the hips to lower back into the chair, stopping a few inches short of the seat. Your thighs should be parallel to the floor.

4. Stay in this isometric hold position for 5-30 seconds, depending on your comfort level. Keep your torso upright and look directly ahead.

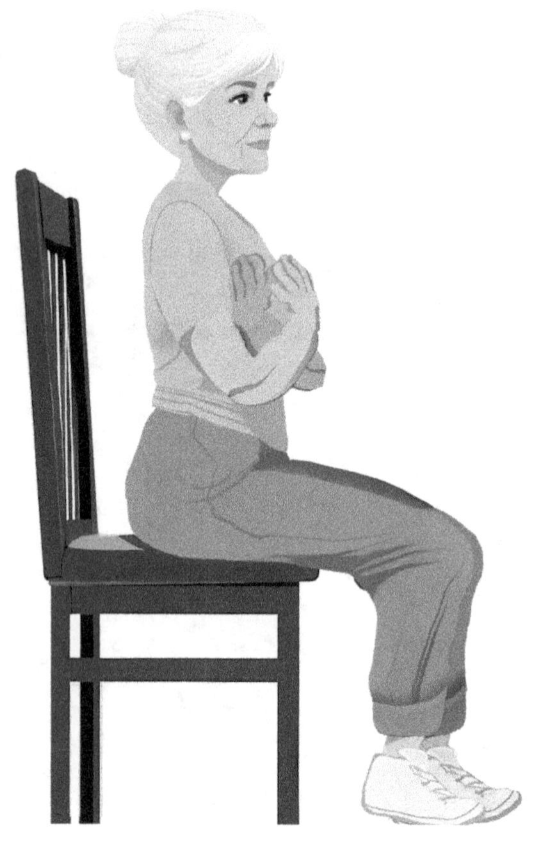
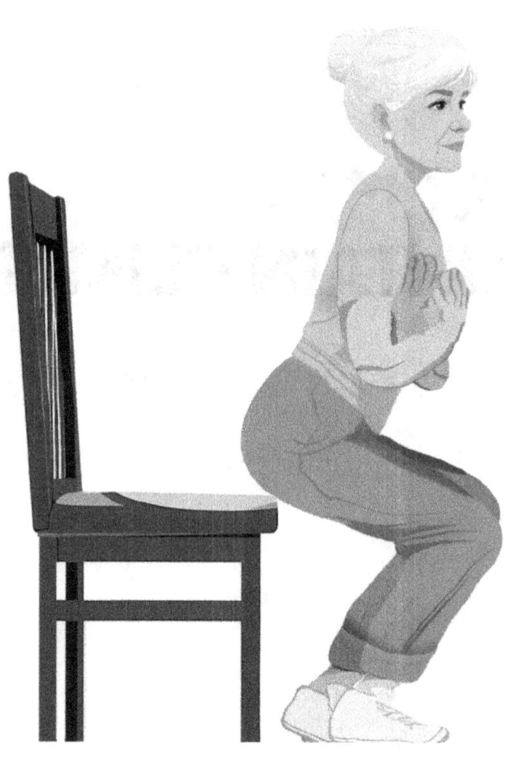

EXERCISE 2
REVERSE CHAIR WARRIOR POSE HOLD

1. Sit upright with your feet wide apart.

2. Turn your left foot out while your right foot straightens outward to the side.

3. Bend your left knee to a 90-degree angle while keeping your right leg straight. Keep your torso facing forward and gaze over your left hand.

4. Extend your left arm overhead as you tilt your torso to the right, and bring the right arm down your leg as far as you comfortably can.

5. Hold the warrior pose for 10-30 seconds, depending on your comfort level.

6. Repeat on the other side.

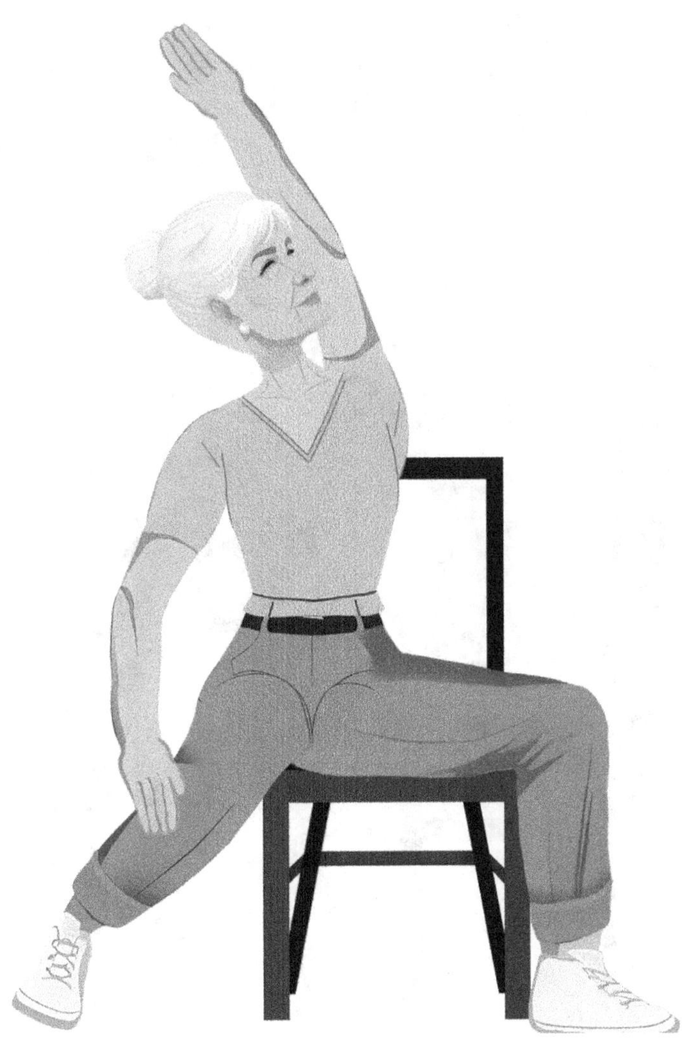

EXERCISE 3
CHAIR BRIDGE HOLD

1. Sit all on the edge of your chair with your hands on the armrests.

2. Push your heels onto the floor as you push through the triceps to lift yourself out of the seated position.

3. Hold this position for a count of 5.

4. Return to the starting position.

5. Perform 5 repetitions of this exercise.

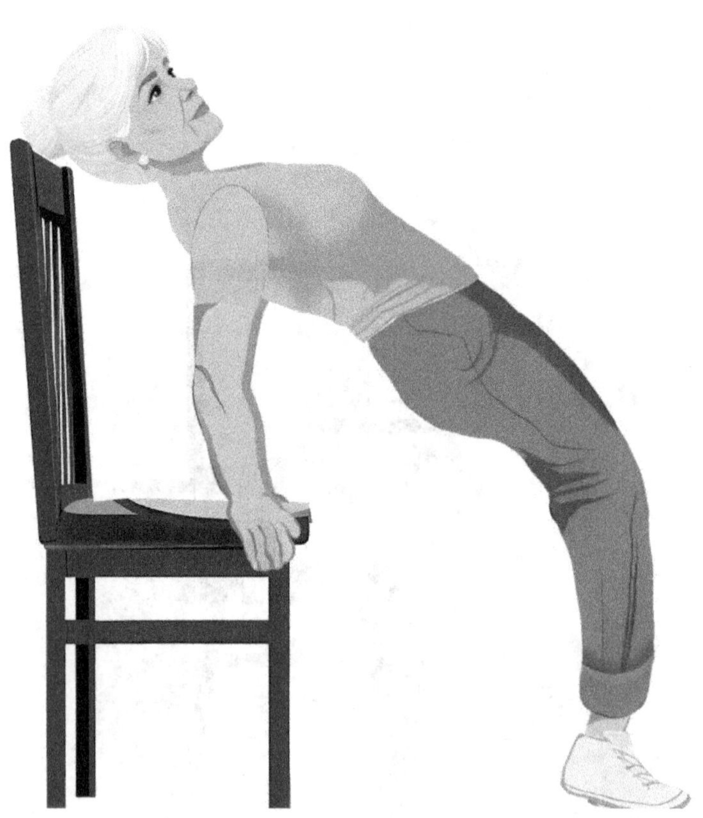

EXERCISE 4
CHAIR PLANK HOLD

1. Stand facing the chair and place your hands on the armrests.

2. Step your feet back until your body forms a 45-degree angle to the floor. Your body should form a straight line from head to heel.

3. Tense your core, legs, and arms.

4. Hold this position for 5-30 seconds, depending on your comfort level.

5. Rest for 2-3 minutes, then repeat these four exercises.

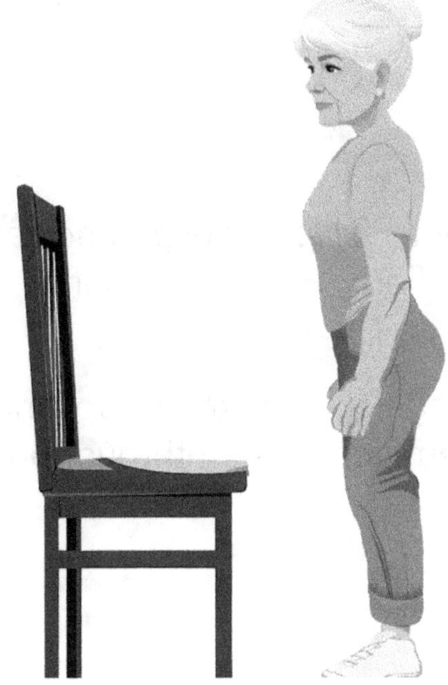

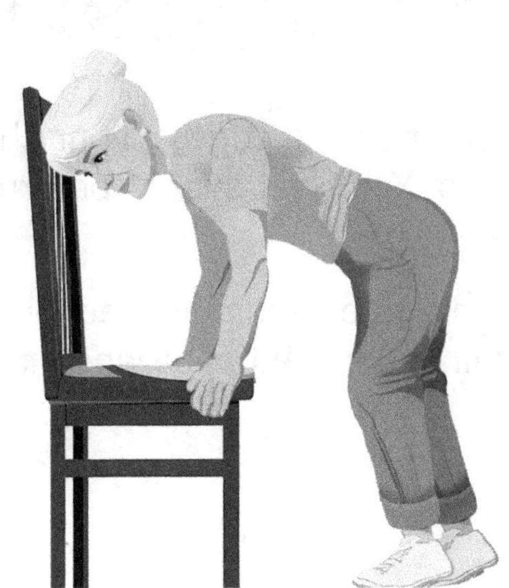

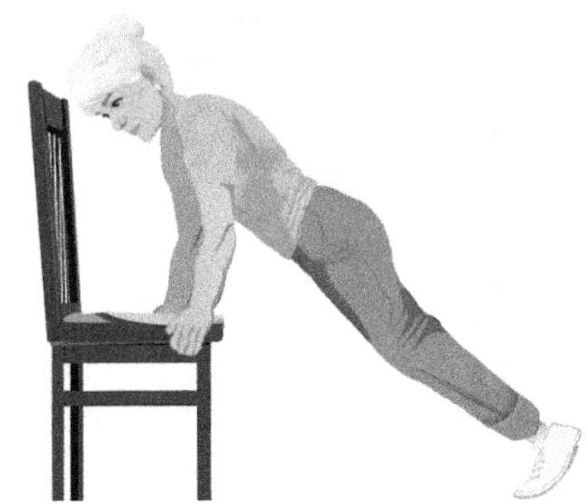

DAY 14 Active Recovery

Today, you will take a break from your chair yoga exercises. Instead, you should go for a 30-minute walk. If possible, get out into nature to enjoy the sights and sounds around you. Practice mindful meditation as you become present in the moment and aware of all your senses.

If your lack of mobility prevents you from doing the above, I recommend that you do several 5-minute sessions of seated marching throughout the day.

SEATED MARCHING

1. Sit upright on the edge of your chair with your shoulder blades pulled back and your chest up. Your feet should be firmly planted on the floor. Place your hands on your thighs.

2. Begin a seated marching action by alternately bringing your knees up and down. Maintain a constant pace, ensuring that your torso remains upright throughout.

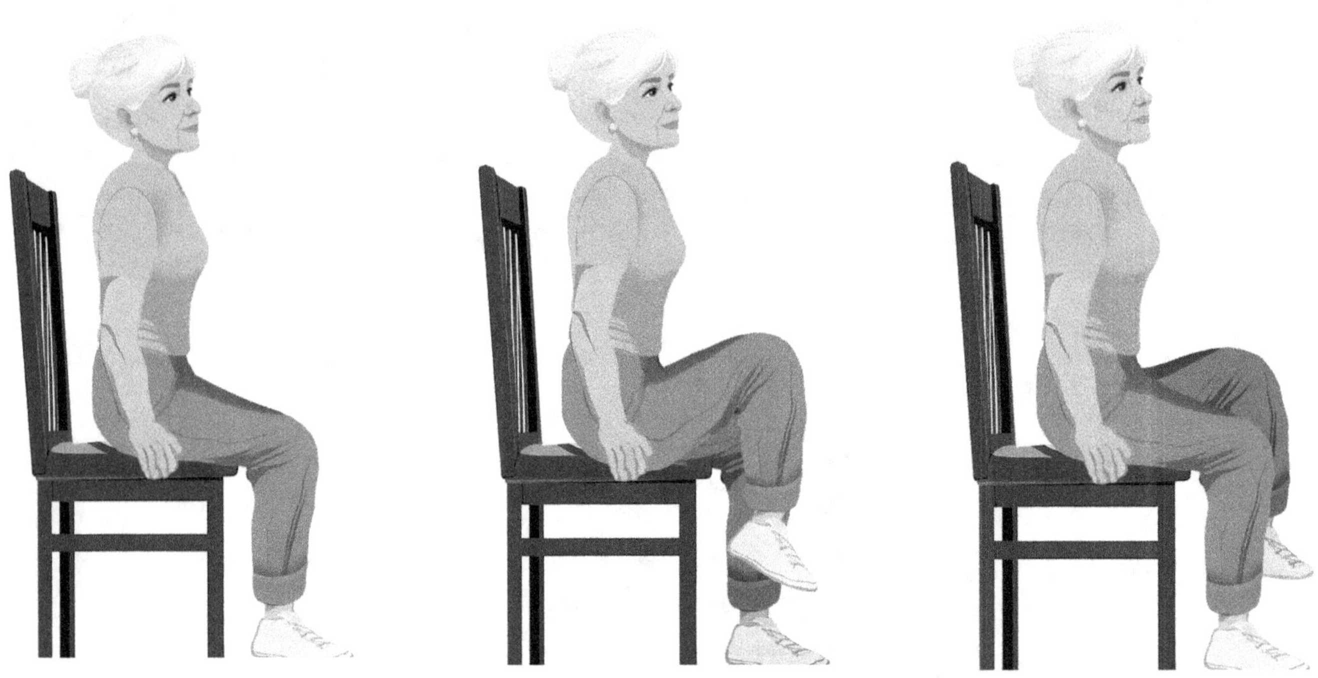

STRENGTH
UPPER BODY

This week, we introduce chair yoga exercises for the upper body. Increasing the strength of your chest, back, shoulder, and arm muscles will enhance your overall posture, stability, and range of motion. These targeted exercises promote flexibility, improve circulation, and alleviate tension in key muscle groups.

You'll also work your lower body and core with a slightly more challenging version of the previous week's sessions.

DAY 15 Upper Body Strength

EXERCISE 1
STEP OUT & PRESS

1. Sit comfortably on the chair with your back straight and feet flat on the floor, hip-width apart. Ensure a stable base and relaxed shoulders.

2. Bring your hands to your mid-chest, palms pressed together. Draw your navel toward your spine to engage your core muscles.

3. Inhale deeply, and as you exhale, step your right foot forward, extending it in front of you. Maintain stability by keeping your weight centered over your hips.

4. Simultaneously, extend both arms overhead in a pressing motion. Keep your palms facing each other, and fully extend your arms without locking the elbows.

5. Lower and repeat.

6. Do fifteen reps of this exercise.

EXERCISE 2
CHEST FLIES

1. Sit upright in your chair with your shoulder blades pulled back and your chest expanded.

2. Take a deep breath as you extend your straightened arms to your sides at shoulder level. Feel the stretch through your chest muscles.

3. Exhale as you slowly bring your arms together to touch your fingertips at chest level.

4. Squeeze your chest tightly in this position.

5. Perform 15 repetitions of this exercise.

EXERCISE 3
LOWER BACK STRETCH

1. Sit on the edge of your chair with your feet firmly planted on the floor. Interlace your fingers in front of your chest.

2. Round your back as you lower your chest toward your knees to extend the spine fully.

3. Now, arch your back by pulling your spine in, tightening your core, and pulling your shoulder blades back to return to an upright position.

4. Perform 15 repetitions of this exercise.

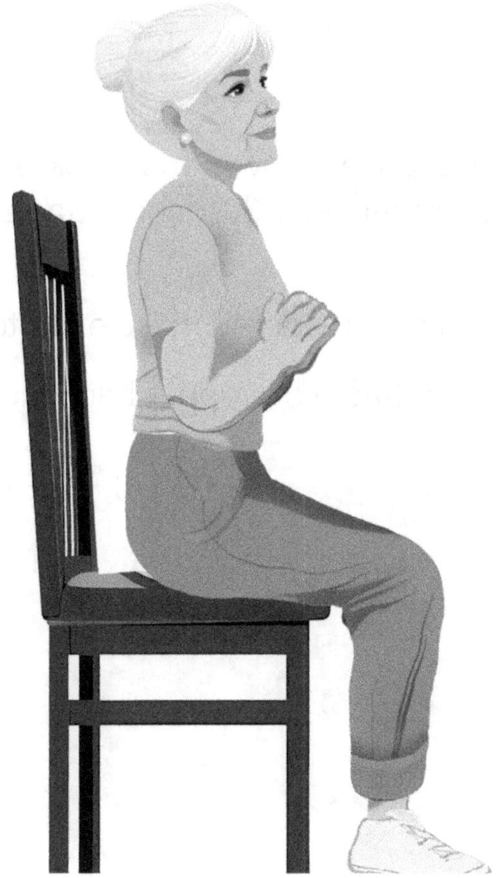

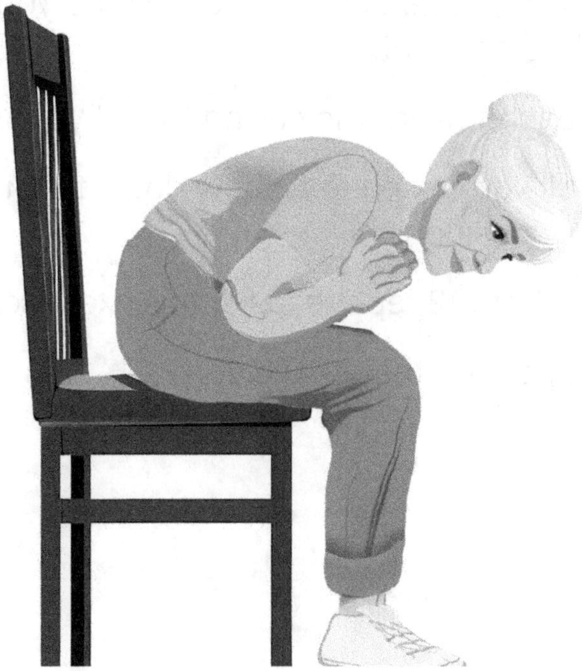

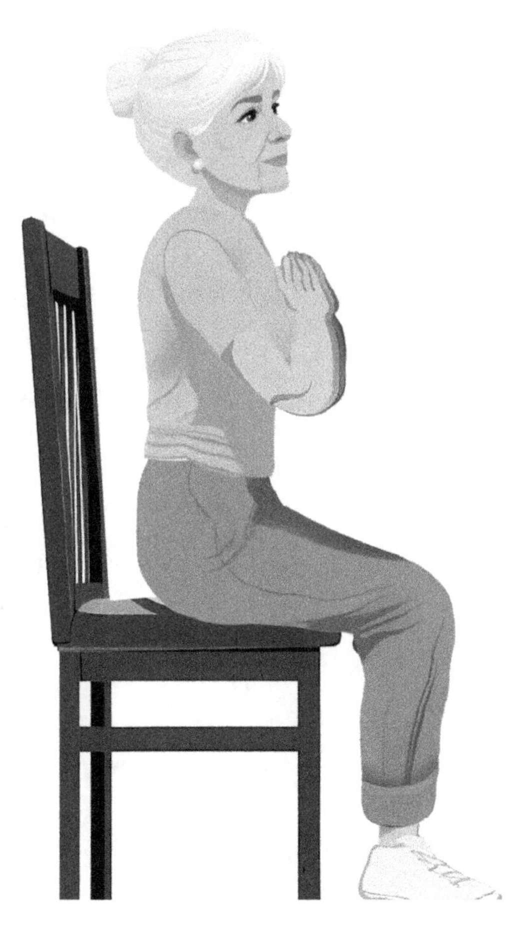

EXERCISE 4
LAT PULL INS

1. Sit upright in your chair with your shoulder blades pulled down and back and feet firmly planted on the floor. Extend your right arm overhead at a 30-degree angle to the shoulder joint.

2. Reach toward the ceiling to feel your upper back (latissimus dorsi) muscle stretching.

3. Pull your extended elbow down to touch your hip. Contract your upper back muscle in this position.

4. Perform 12 repetitions of this exercise.

5. Repeat on the other side.

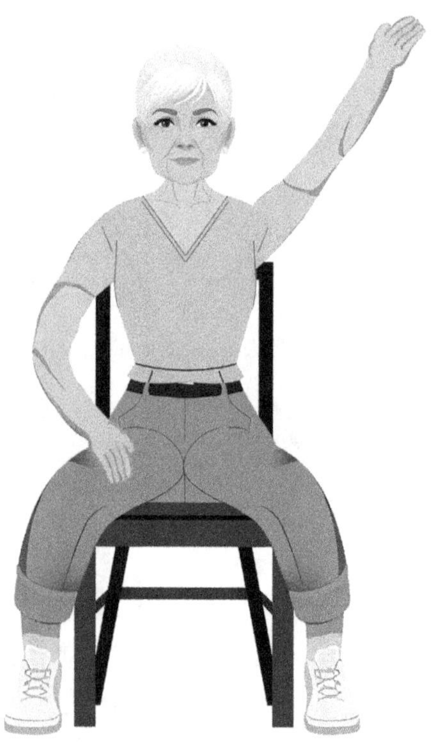
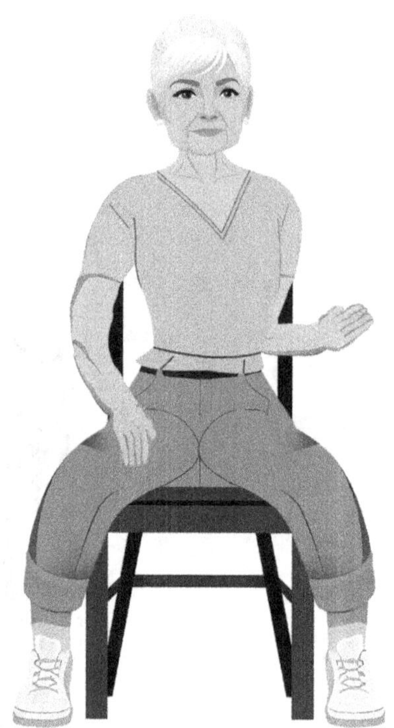

EXERCISE 5
CHAIR DIPS

1. Sit on the edge of your chair with your hands on the edge of the seat, palms down. Extend your legs out in front of you, feet together.

2. Straighten your arms to lift your butt off the chair.

3. Scoot slightly forward so your butt is off the chair.

4. Bend at the elbows to lower your body toward the floor. Keep going until your elbows are at right angles.

5. Push through your triceps (back of the upper arms) to return to the start position.

6. Rest for 2-3 minutes, then repeat these five exercises.

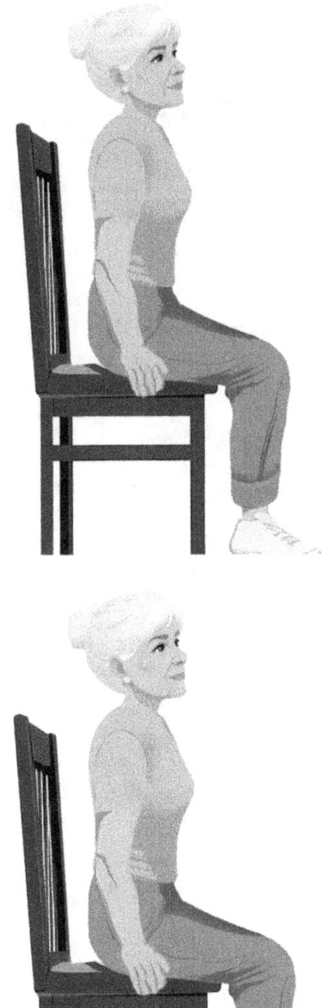

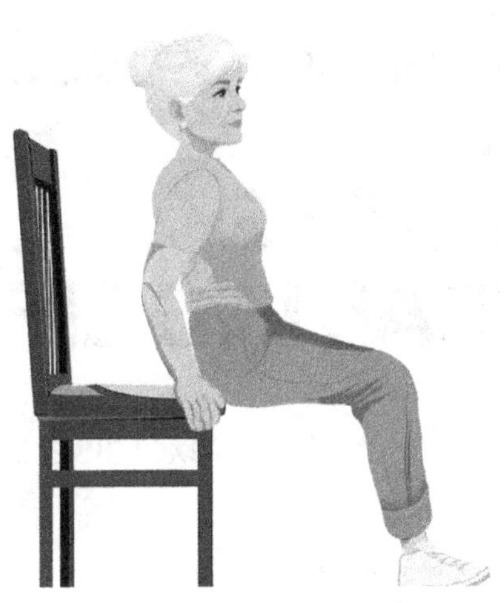

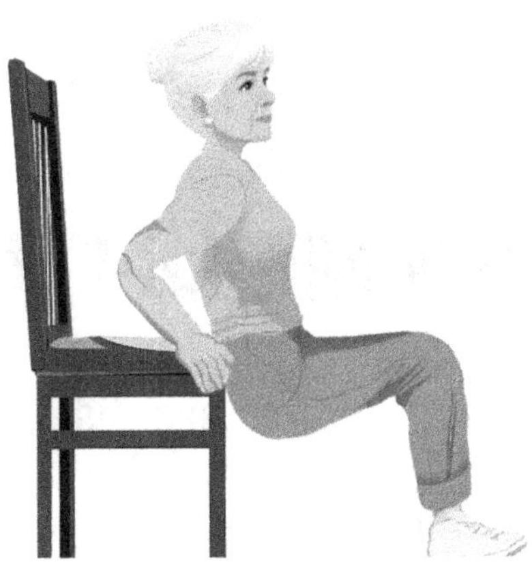

DAY 16 Lower Body Strength

EXERCISE 1
LEG EXTENSION

Do 15 repetitions of this exercise on each leg.

EXERCISE 2
LEG DRAG

Do 15 repetitions of this exercise on each leg.

EXERCISE 3
LATERAL LEG LIFT

Do 15 repetitions of this exercise on each leg.

EXERCISE 4
SIT & STAND

Do 5 repetitions of this exercise.

EXERCISE 5
SEATED MOUNTAIN

Do 10 repetitions of this exercise.

Rest for 2-3 minutes, then repeat these five exercises.

DAY 17 Core Strength

EXERCISE 1
CHAIR SPINAL TWIST

Do 15 repetitions of this exercise.

EXERCISE 2
CHAIR GODDESS TWIST

Do 15 repetitions of this exercise.

EXERCISE 3
CHAIR BOAT POSE

Do 12 repetitions of this exercise.

EXERCISE 4
MOUNTAIN CLIMBER

Do 15 repetitions of this exercise.

EXERCISE 5
PIKE PULSE

1. Sit on the edge of your chair with your feet extended in front of you. Ensure your back is straight and your hands are resting on your thighs or lap.

2. Activate your core muscles by drawing your navel toward your spine.

3. Inhale as you extend both arms forward at shoulder height, parallel to the floor. Keep your palms facing each other, creating a straight line from your fingertips through your spine.

4. Exhale and hinge at the hips, leaning forward with a straight back. Maintain core engagement to support the movement.

5. Once you reach the maximum comfortable stretch forward, initiate small pulsing movements by contracting and releasing your core muscles. Pulse for ten repetitions, maintaining control and a steady pace.

6. Inhale as you return to an upright seated position.

7. Rest for 2-3 minutes, then repeat these five exercises.

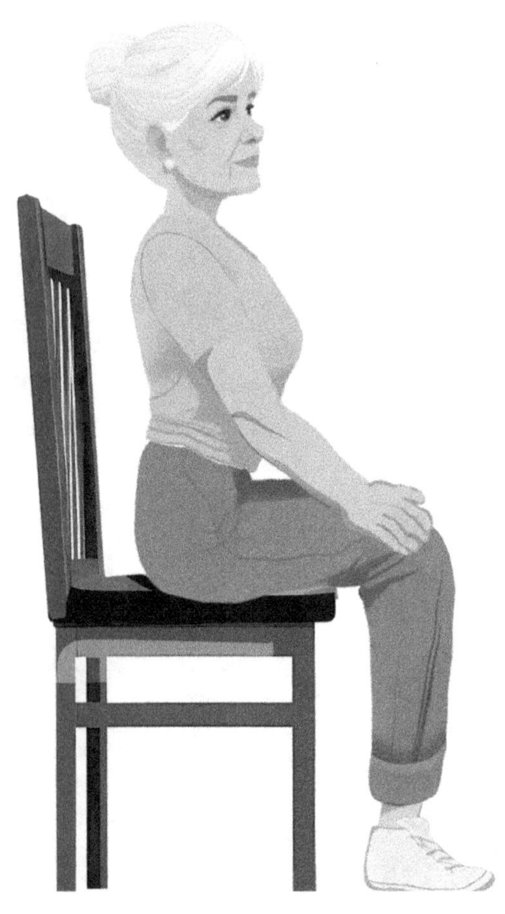
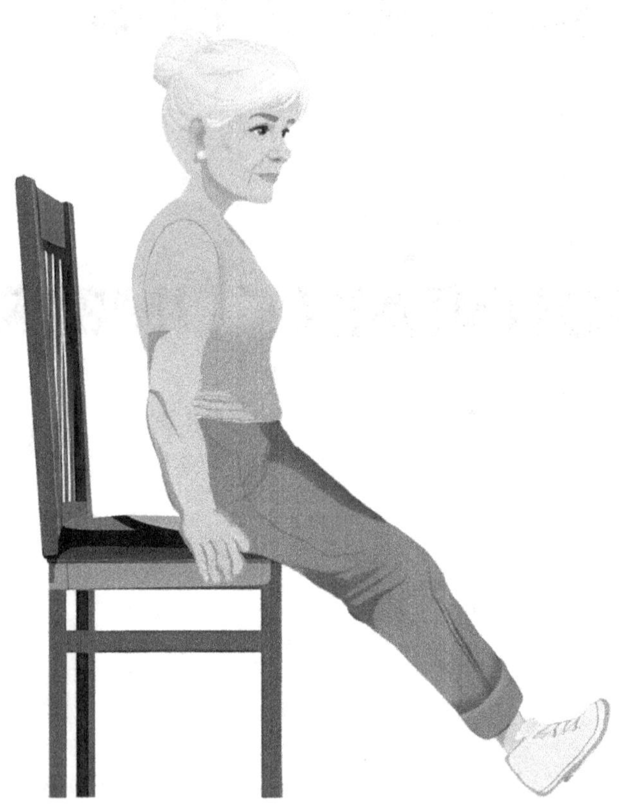

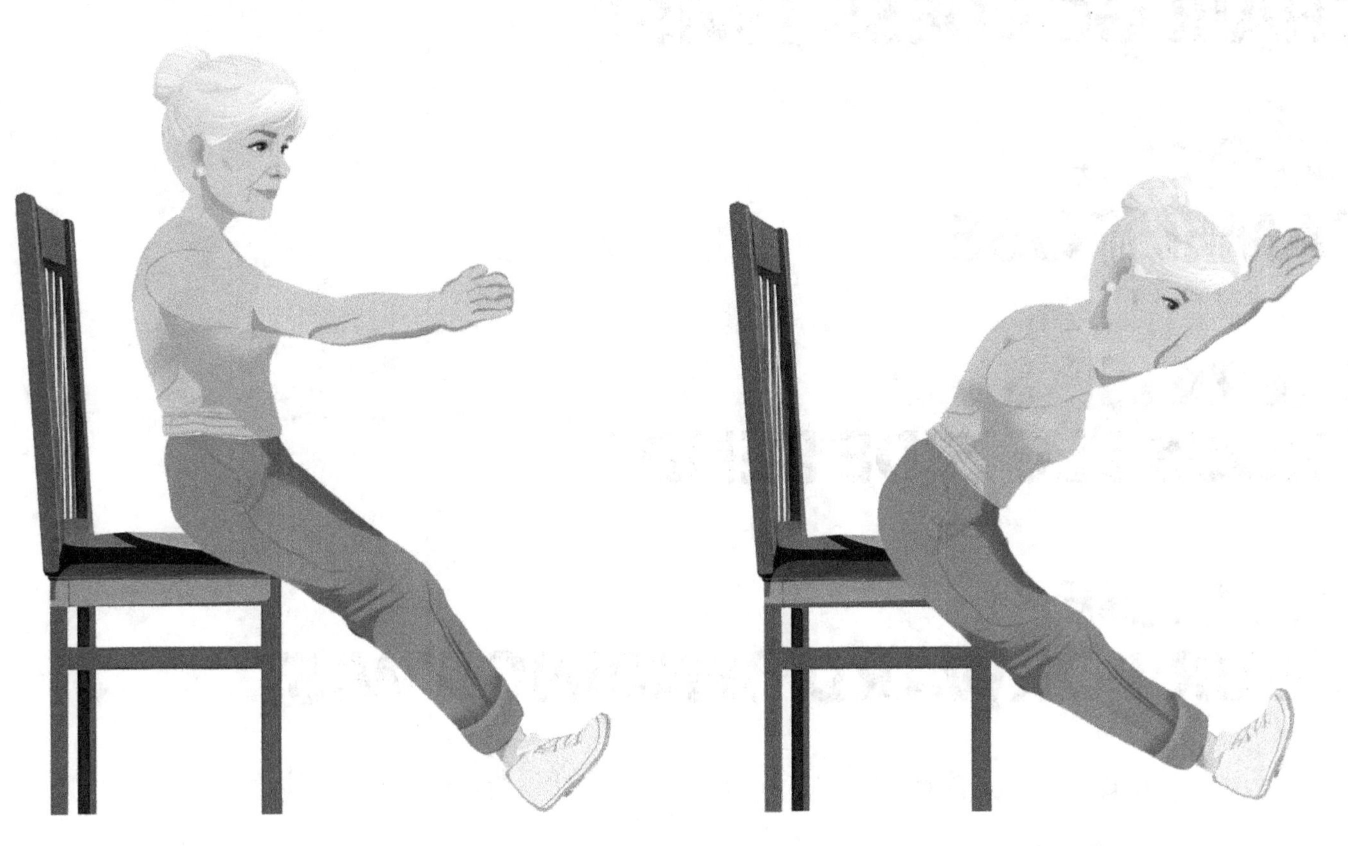

DAY 18 Spinal Health

EXERCISE 1
CHAIR GODDESS TWIST

EXERCISE 2
CAMEL POSE

EXERCISE 3
CROSS LEG SIDE BEND

EXERCISE 4
CHAIR FORWARD BENDING TWIST

1. Sit with your back straight and your feet flat on the floor hip-width apart.

2. Inhale deeply as you lengthen your spine, sitting up tall. Imagine your head reaching toward the ceiling.

3. Exhale as you twist your torso to the right and down, bringing your left hand down to the floor. Simultaneously, lift your right hand toward the ceiling.

4. Hold the twist for a count of five, feeling the stretch along the spine. Keep your shoulders relaxed and your neck aligned with your spine as you look up toward your extended hand.

5. Inhale as you return to the center, bringing your spine back to a neutral position.

6. Repeat on the other side.

7. Do 8 repeats of this exercise on each side.

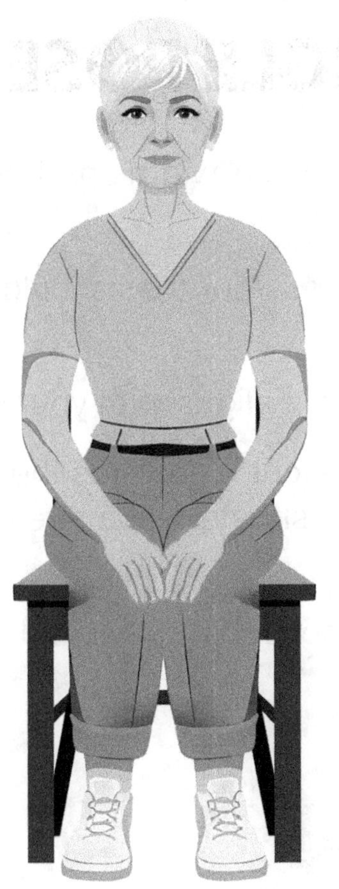 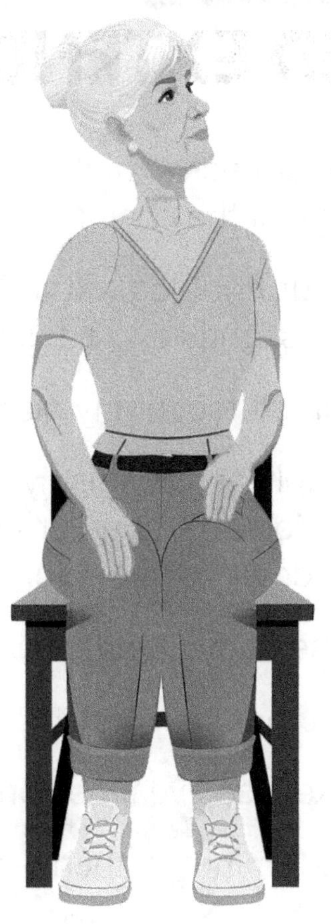

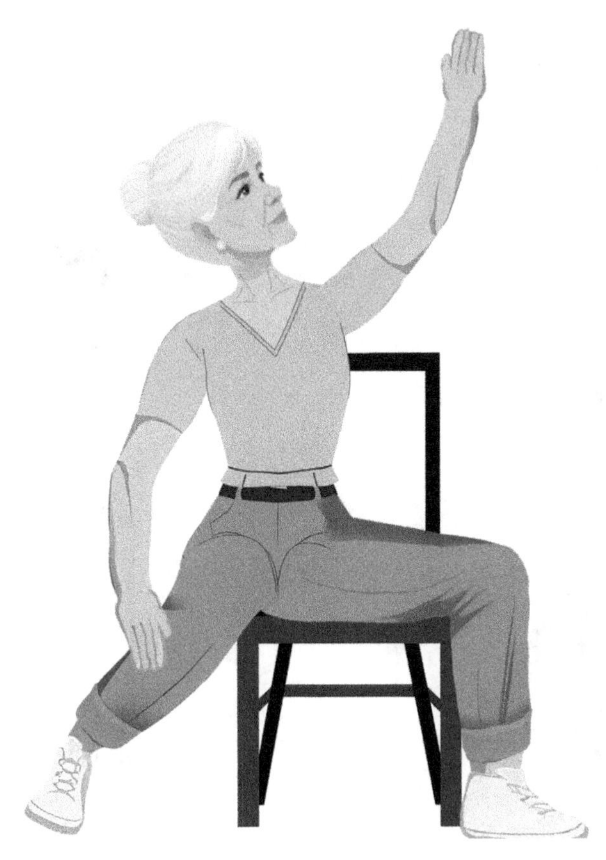

EXERCISE 5
SEATED EXTENDED SIDE ANGLE POSE

1. Sit with your back straight and your feet flat on the floor, hip-width apart. Slide forward to the edge of the chair.

2. Extend your right leg out to the side, keeping it straight. Your toes should be pointing forward or slightly angled upwards.

3. Keep your left foot firmly planted on the floor, ensuring it aligns with your hip.

4. Inhale deeply as you raise your right arm overhead, reaching towards the ceiling. Rest your right forearm on your right thigh. Your right side should feel a stretch from your fingertips down to your hip.

5. Hold the seated extended side angle pose for fifteen seconds.

6. Repeat on the other side.

7. Do this exercise five times on each side.

8. Rest for 2-3 minutes, then repeat these five exercises.

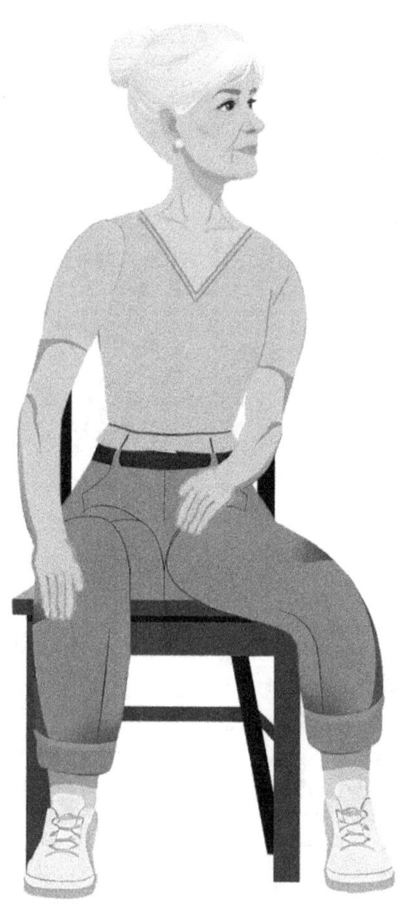
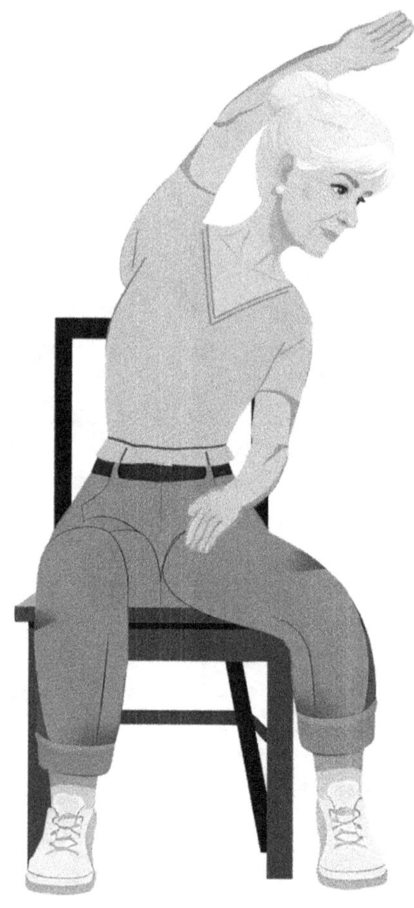

Upper Body Strength

EXERCISE 1
STEP OUT & PRESS

Perform 15 repetitions of this exercise.

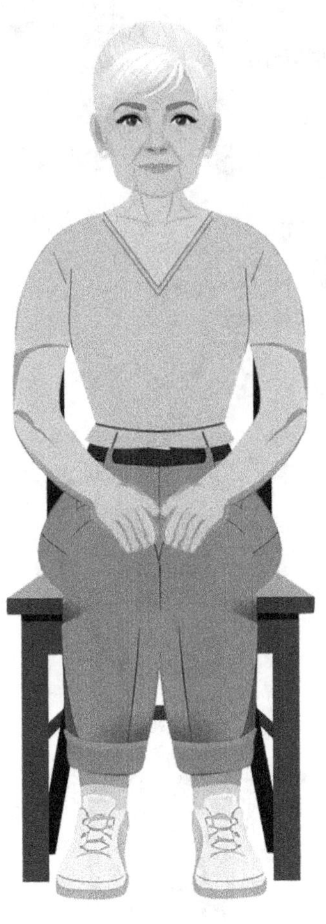
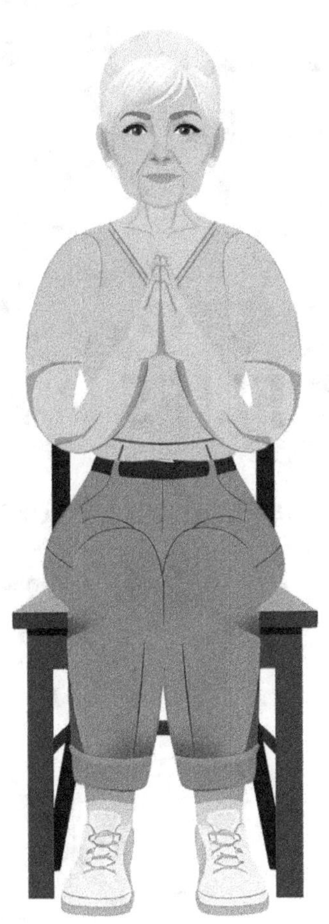

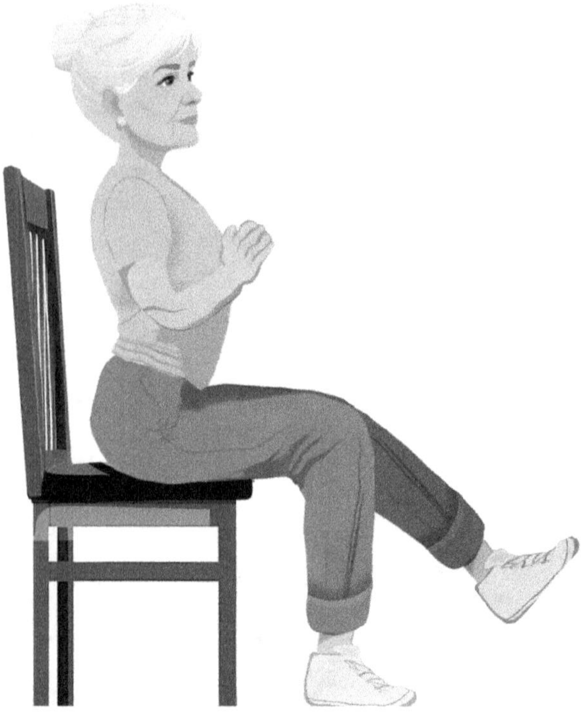

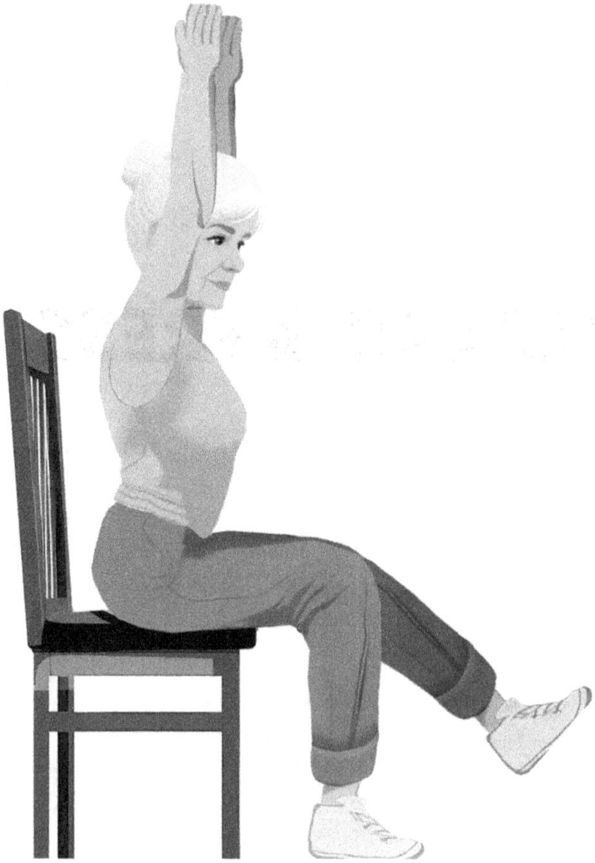

EXERCISE 2: CHEST FLIES

Perform 15 repetitions of this exercise.

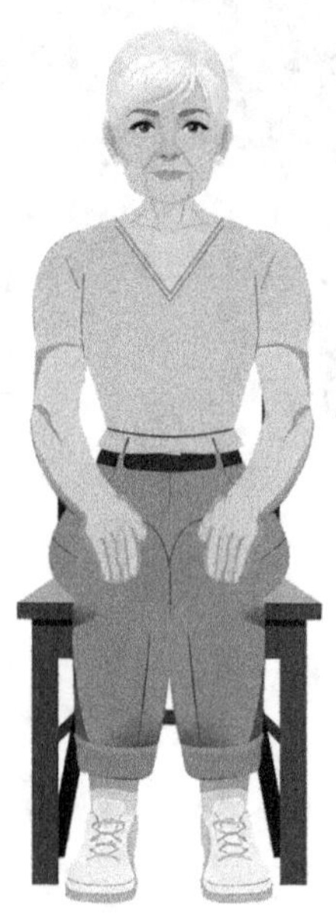 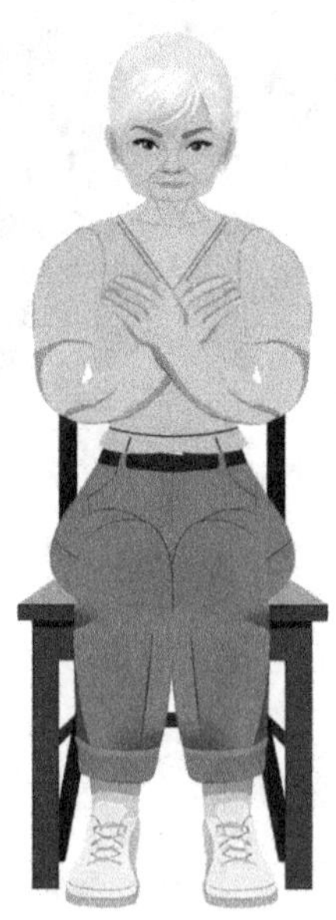

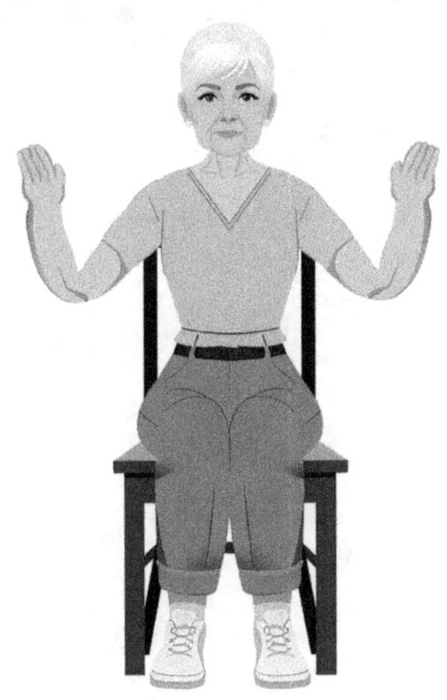

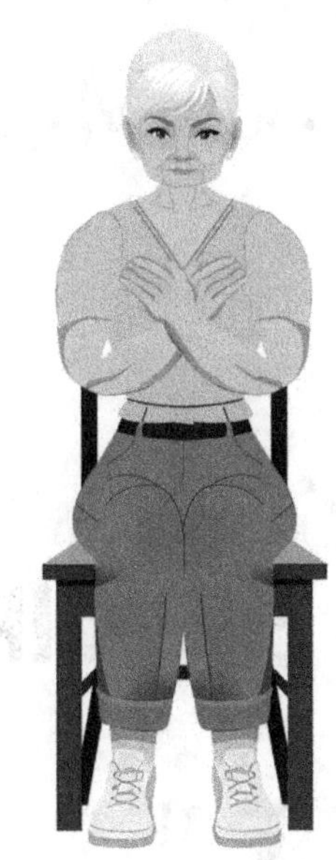

EXERCISE 3
LOWER BACK STRETCH

Perform 15 repetitions of this exercise.

EXERCISE 4
LAT PULL INS

Perform 12 repetitions on this exercise

EXERCISE 5
CHAIR DIPS

Perform 15 repetitions on this exercise

Rest for 2-3 minutes, then repeat these five exercises.

DAY 20 Hip Mobility

EXERCISE 1
SEATED HIP CIRCLES

EXERCISE 2
EAGLE TWIST

EXERCISE 3
FORWARD FOLD

EXERCISE 4
REVERSE TABLE TOP

1. Position yourself side-on to your chair and assume a table-top position with your shoulders on the chair, your torso straight and your knees bent at 90-degrees.

2. Extend your arms overhead and then bend the elbows, so that your hands are pointing to the floor.

3. Breathe out as you open your chest and expand your ribcage.

4. Hold this position for 15 seconds.

5. Perform 5 repetitions of this exercise.

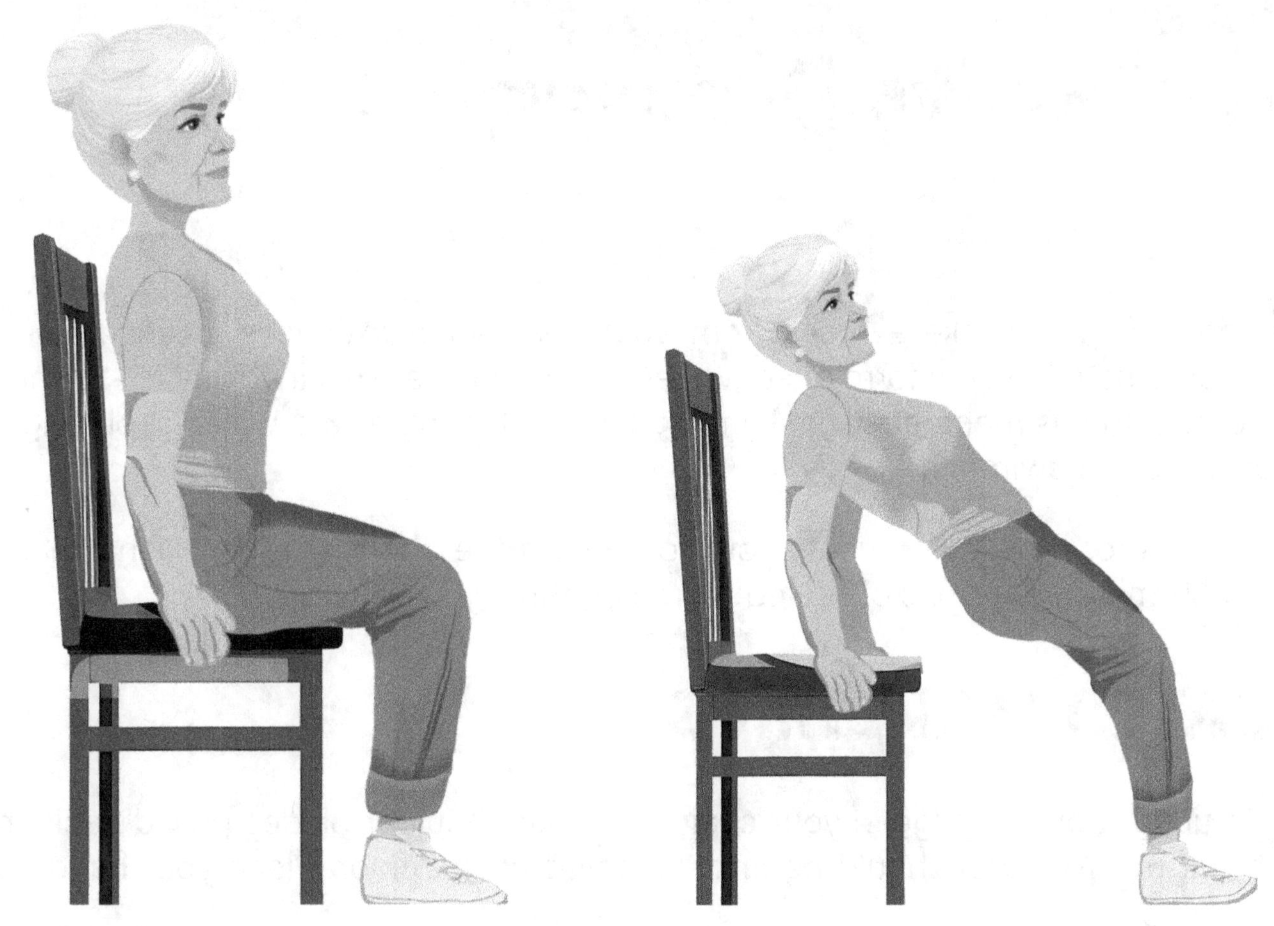

EXERCISE 5
LATERAL LEG LIFT

Active Recovery

Today, you will take a break from your chair yoga exercises. Instead, you should participate in some form of active recovery exercise. This involves 20-30 minutes of movement that is moderately challenging for you. Examples are walking, playing a game of pickleball, or swimming.

If your lack of mobility prevents you from doing the above, I recommend that you do several 5-minute sessions of seated marching throughout the day.

SEATED MARCHING

1. Sit upright on the edge of your chair with your shoulder blades pulled back and your chest up. Your feet should be firmly planted on the floor. Place your hands on your thighs.

2. Begin a seated marching action by alternately bringing your knees up and down. Maintain a constant pace, ensuring that your torso remains upright throughout.

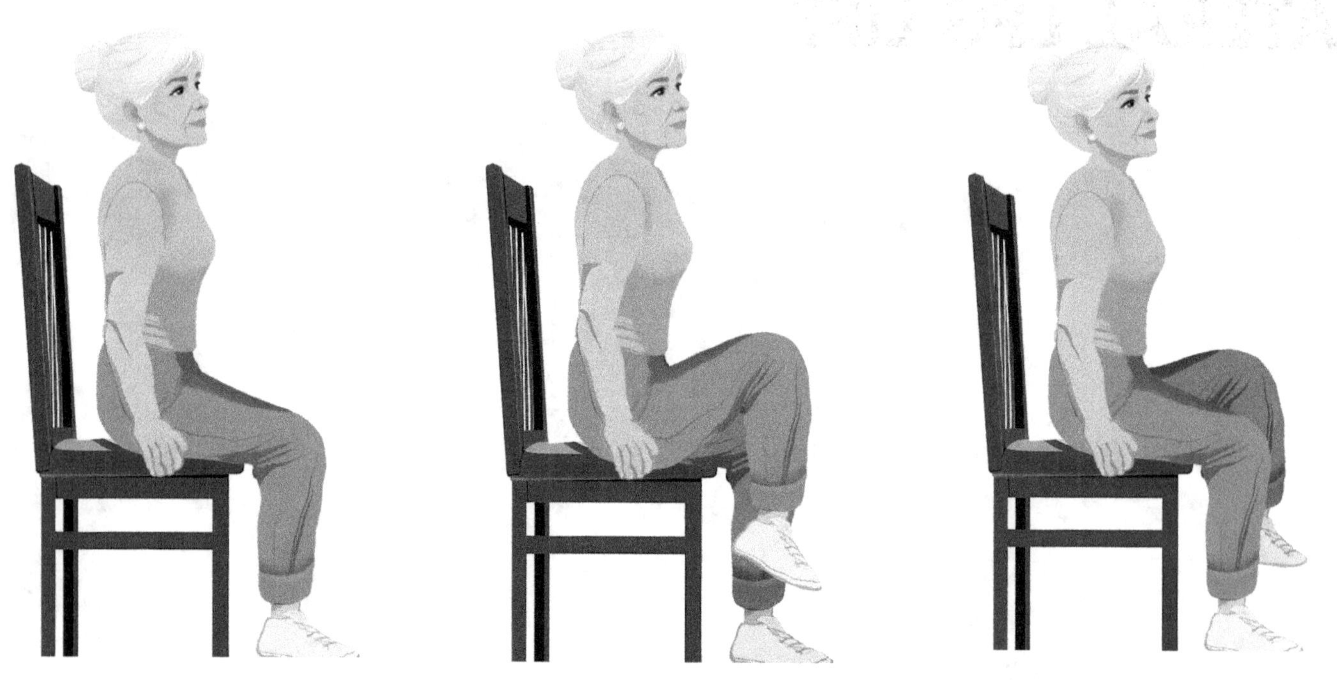

FUNCTIONAL MOVEMENT

In this, the final week of the Chair Yoga Challenge, we focus on movements that involve full-body integration. In previous weeks, we've given attention to different parts of the body on different days. This has been necessary to build a foundation of strength and stability.

Now, we're ready to challenge the body more functionally by incorporating movements that engage multiple muscle groups simultaneously. This holistic approach strengthens the body and improves coordination, balance, and overall physical performance.

DAY 22 Functional Movement 1

EXERCISE 1
CHAIR WARRIOR

1. Sit upright with your feet firmly planted on the ground.

2. Slide your right leg to the side of the chair so it is side-on to your body.

3. Move your left hip across so it is free of the chair, and extend that leg out laterally to form a 30-degree angle. Keep your torso upright with your shoulder directly above your hips.

4. Bring your arms up and out at shoulder level.

5. Turn your head to the right.

6. Hold this pose for 15 seconds.

7. Repeat on the other side.

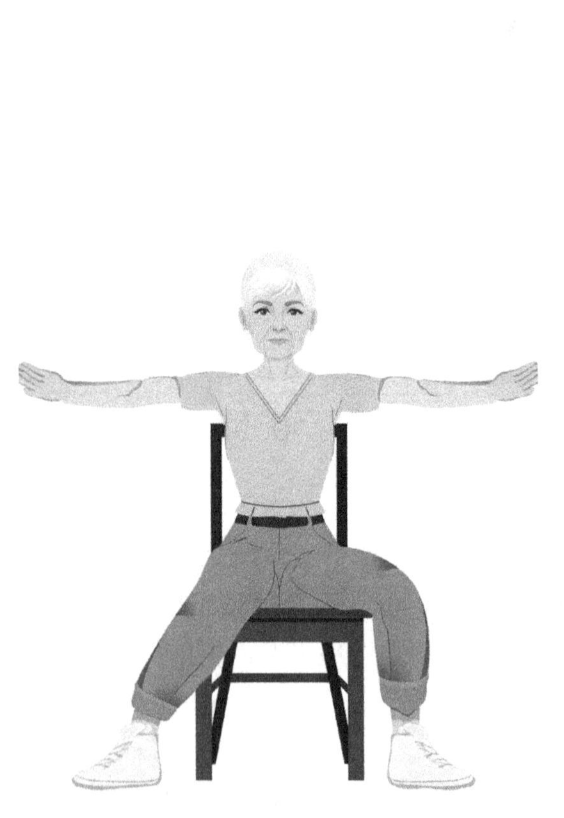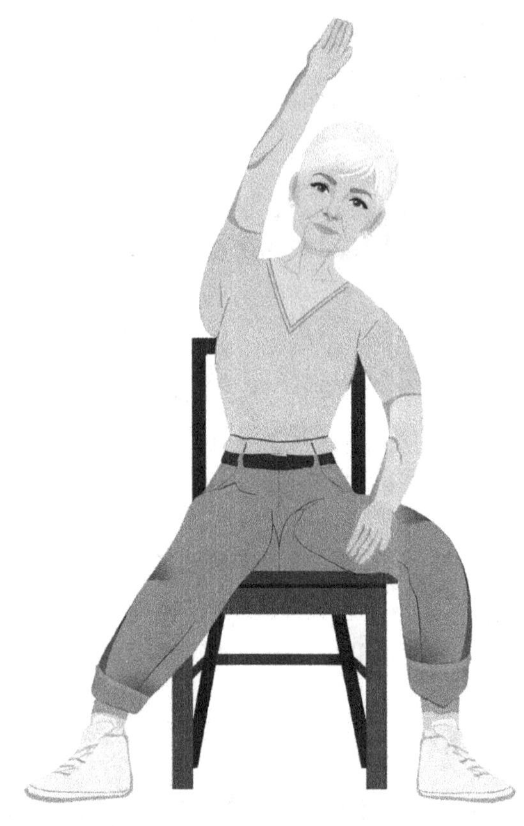

EXERCISE 2
CHAIR REVERSE WARRIOR

EXERCISE 3
REVOLVED HEAD TO KNEE POSE

1. Sit with your back straight and your feet flat on the floor, hip-width apart.

2. Scoot forward until you are sitting on the edge of the chair, allowing space behind you.

3. Extend your right leg straight in front.

4. Extend your right leg straight out to the side, keeping it on the floor. Flex your foot to engage the muscles in your right leg.

5. Bend your left knee, bringing the sole of your left foot to the inside of your right thigh so

that the lower leg rests on the chair.

6. Inhale deeply as you raise your right arm overhead, reaching towards the ceiling. Keep your palm facing inward.

7. Exhale and twist towards the right.

8. Hold the pose for fifteen seconds.

9. Repeat on the other side.

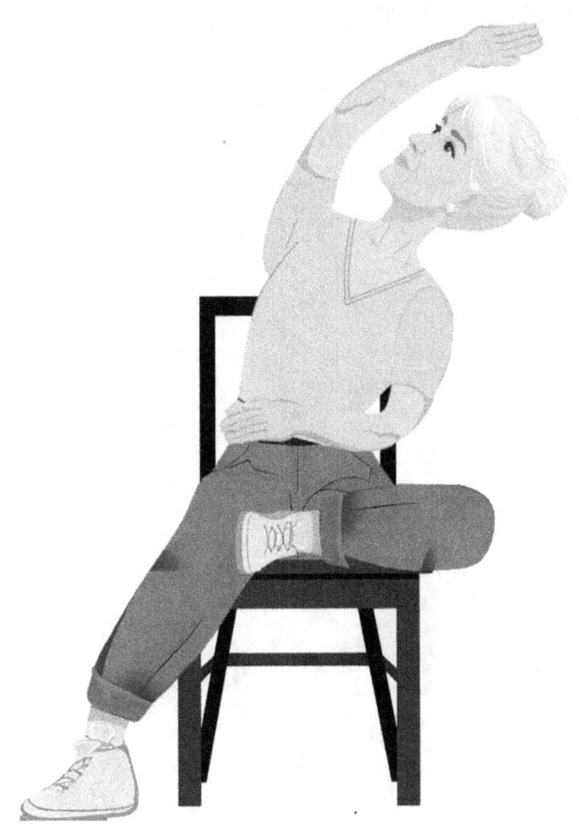

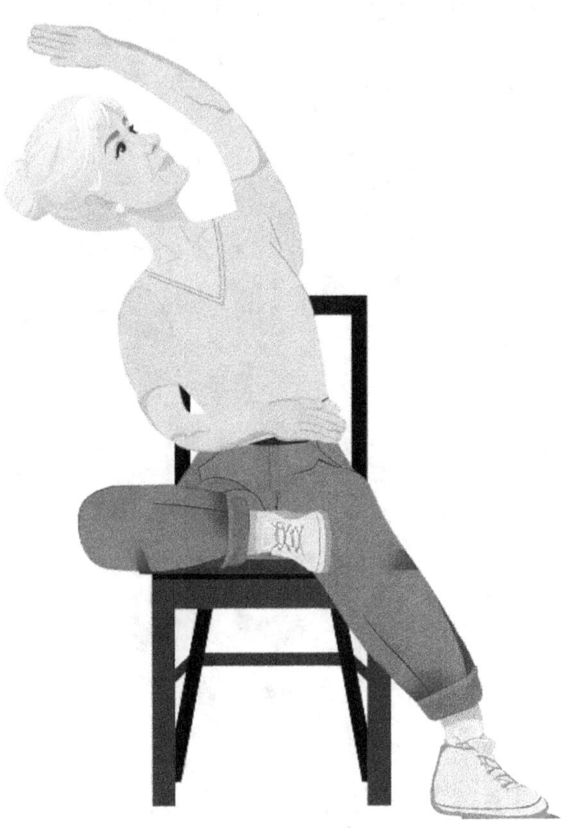

EXERCISE 4
SEATED WARRIOR II

1. Sit on your chair, feet flat on the floor and your left foot in front. Sit tall, engaging your core and keeping your spine straight.

2. Shift your weight onto your left foot, firmly planting it into the ground. Extend your right leg behind you, planting the balls of your feet on the floor.

3. Reach your hands overhead to touch your fingertips above your head. Stretch through your upper back as you hold the pose. Tighten your core muscles to maintain balance and stability. Focus on pulling your navel toward your spine.

4. Hold the Warrior II pose for fifteen to thirty seconds or longer if comfortable. Keep breathing steadily and maintain a strong, controlled posture.

5. Repeat on the other side.

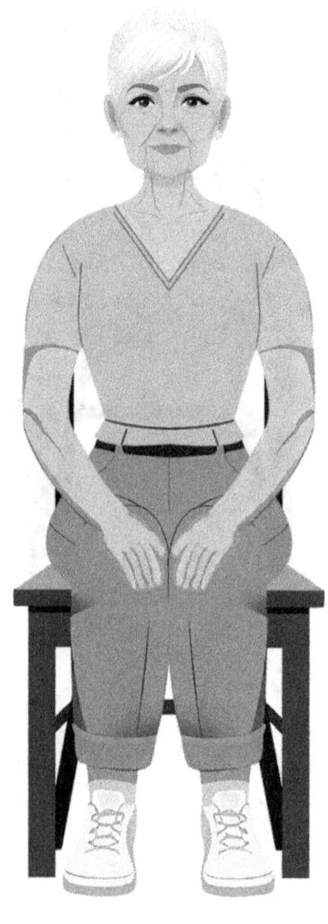
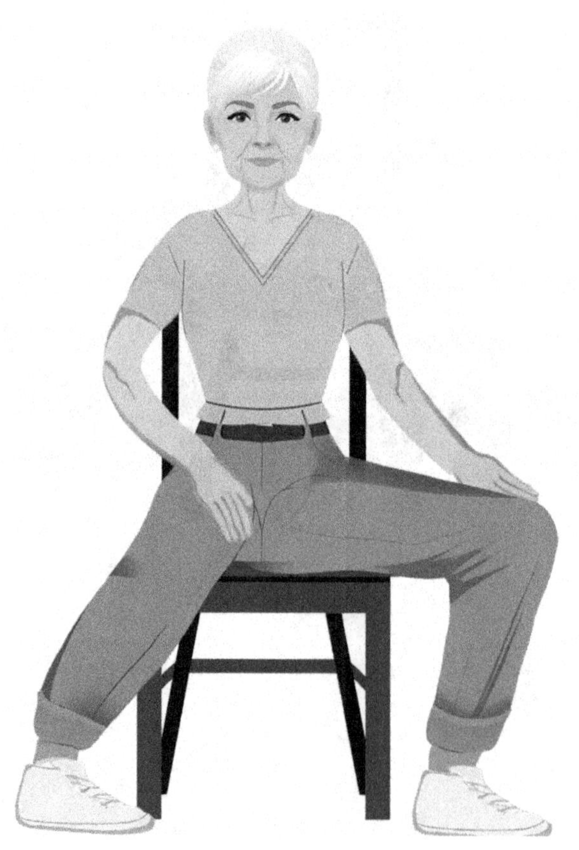

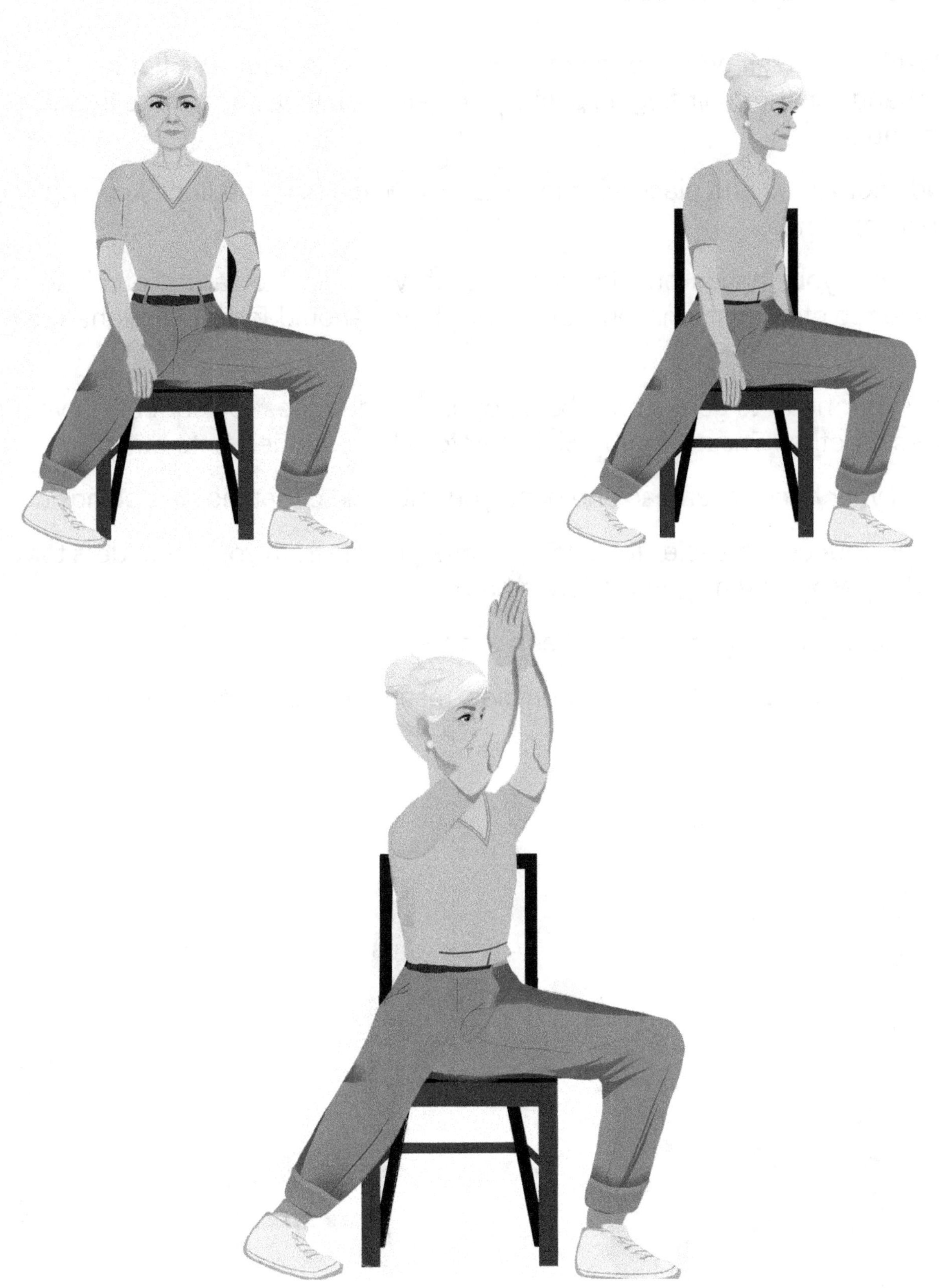

EXERCISE 5
REVERSE TABLE TOP

1. 1. Position yourself on the edge of a sturdy chair with your feet flat on the floor. Place your hands on the chair, fingers pointing toward your feet, and ensure they are shoulder-width apart.

2. Bend your knees and place your feet hip-width apart on the floor, keeping your ankles below your knees.

3. Press into your hands on the chair and lift your hips toward the ceiling, creating a reverse tabletop position. Your torso and thighs should form a straight line parallel to the floor.

4. Allow your head to gently drop back, opening your chest by squeezing your shoulder blades together. Ensure your neck is comfortable and there's no strain.

5. Extend your hands overhead and bend your elbows so that they are alongside your ears.

6. Tighten your core muscles to maintain a straight line from your shoulders to your knees. Avoid excessive arching in the lower back.

7. Hold the extended position for fifteen seconds.

8. Complete three sets of these 5 exercises, resting for 60 seconds between each set.

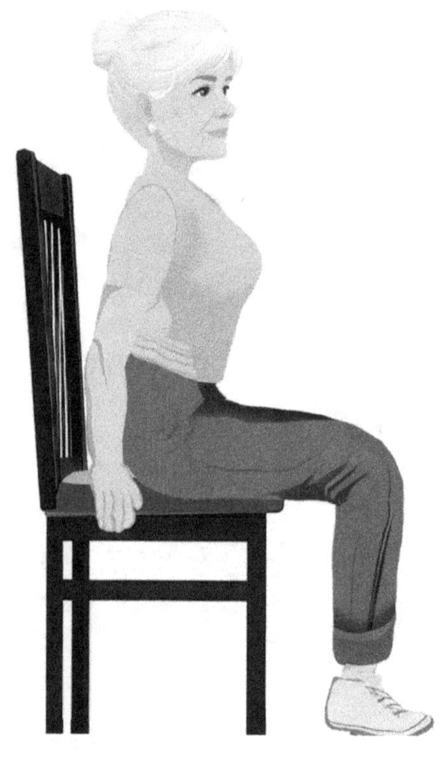
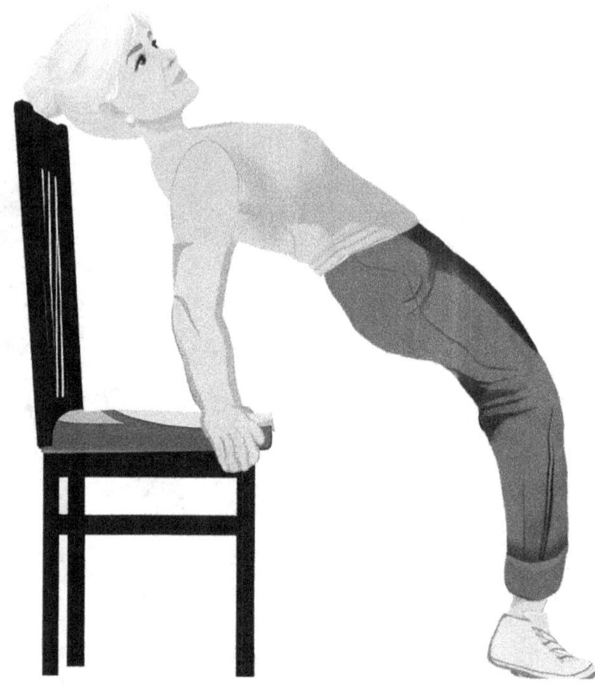

Functional Movement 2

EXERCISE 1
SEATED CHILD'S POSE

1. Sit upright in your chair with your feet flat on the floor.

2. Rest your elbows on your knees and lean forward to elongate your spine. Pull in your lower back and open your shoulder blades.

3. Now, extend your arms directly out before you, reaching forward to stretch the spine further.

4. Hold this position for 15 seconds.

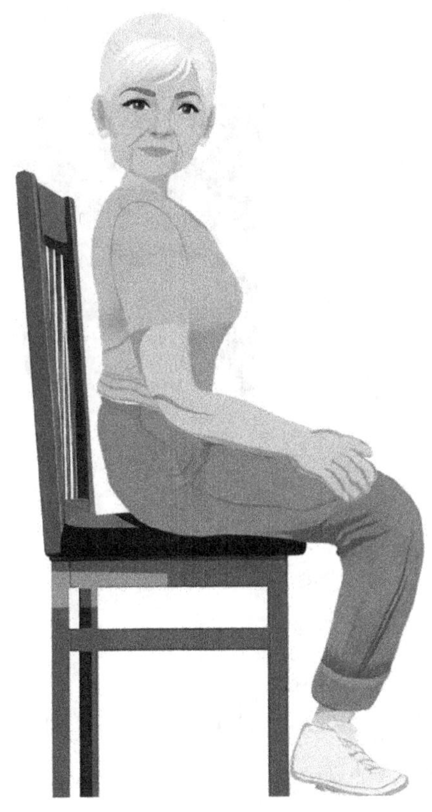
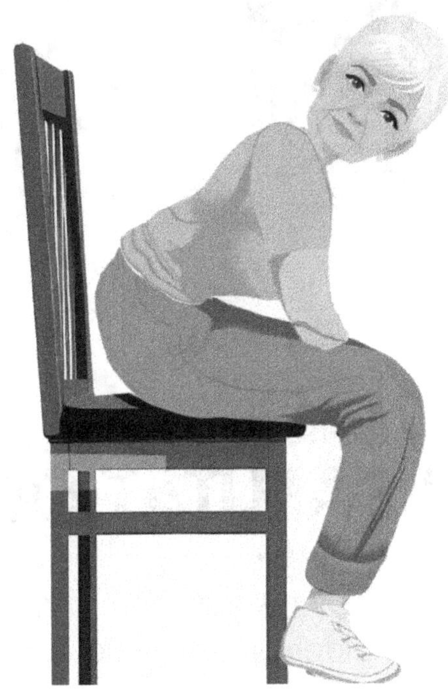

EXERCISE 2
SEATED PIGEON

1. Sit upright in your chair with your butt against the back support.

2. Bring your right ankle over your left knee.

3. Hold the ankle with both hands and gently draw it toward your body. Lengthen your spine and stretch your chest out as you breathe in and look toward the ceiling.

4. Hold this position for five deep breaths through your nose.

5. Repeat on the other side.

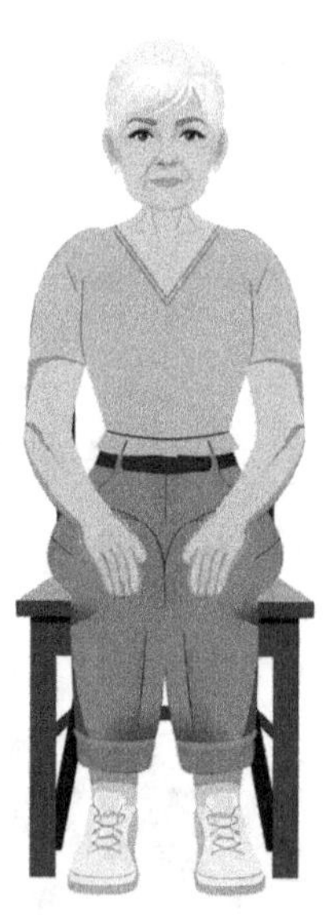 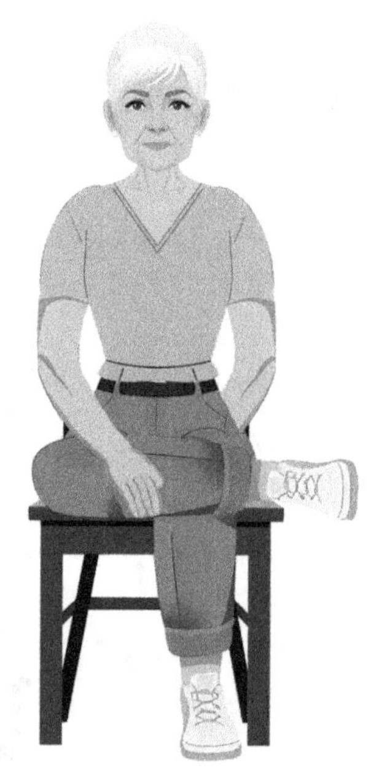 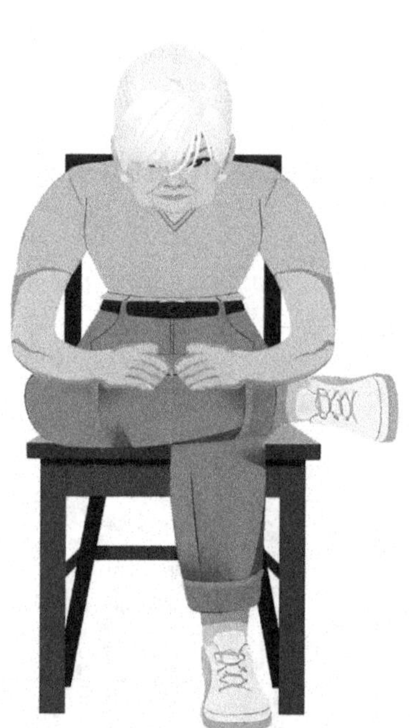

EXERCISE 3
SUN SALUTATION

1. Sit upright with your feet firmly planted on the floor. Maintain an upright torso, with your shoulder blades pulled back and your chest open.

2. Inhale deeply as you reach your arms over to touch your fingertips together overhead.

3. Exhale as you lower your right arm and bend to the right side. Reach your left arm over your head as you feel the stretch through your right side.

4. Repeat on the other side.

5. Now, stretch your arms down as you bring your torso down and stretch forward.

6. Hold this position for 15 seconds.

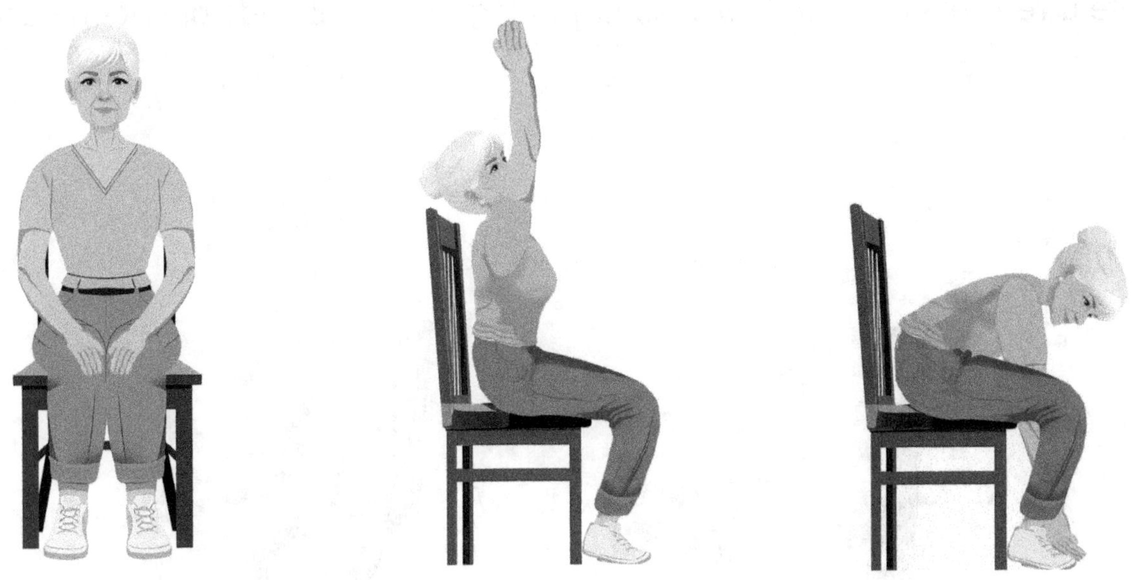

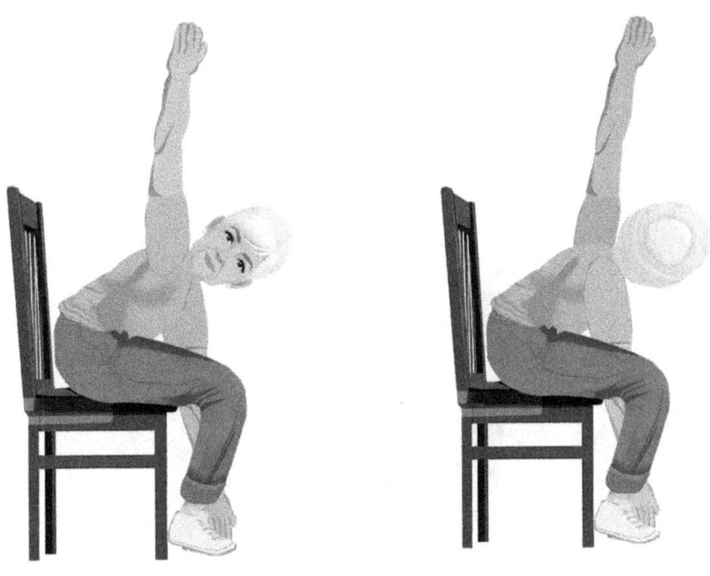

EXERCISE 4
BOAT POSE

EXERCISE 5
SEATED CAT COW

Complete three sets of these 5 exercises, resting for 60 seconds between each set.

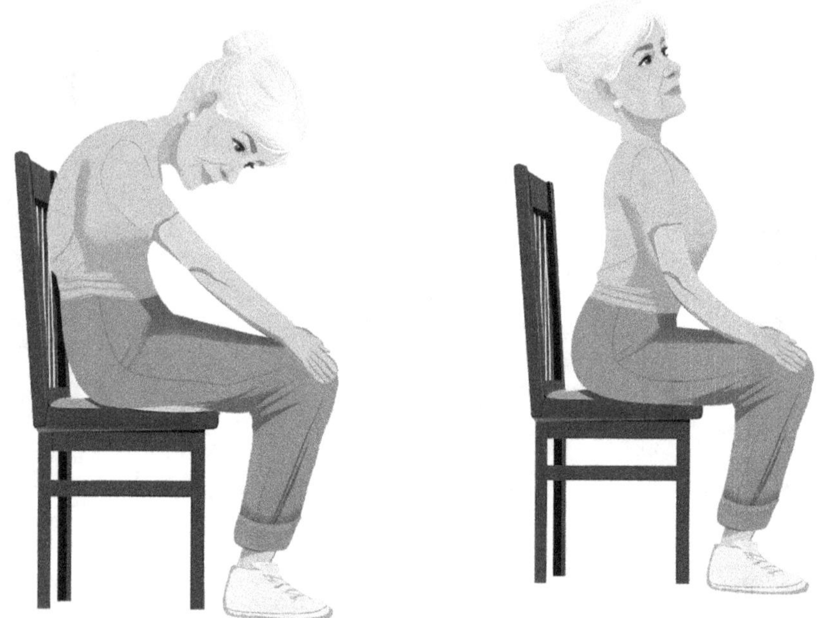

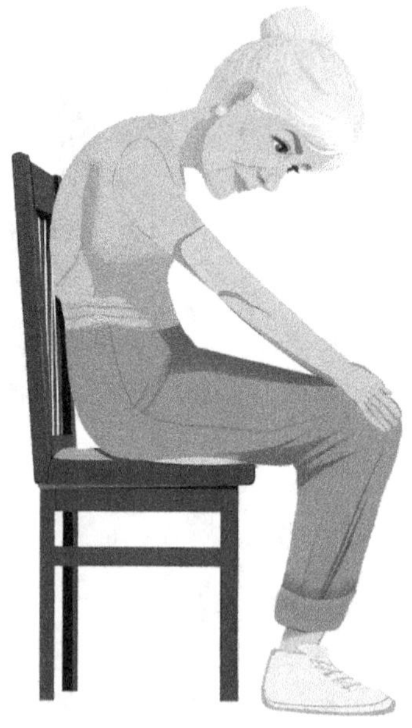

DAY 24 Upper Body Strength

EXERCISE 1
STEP OUT & PRESS

Do fifteen reps of this exercise.

EXERCISE 2
CHEST FLIES

Perform 15 repetitions of this exercise.

EXERCISE 3
LOWER BACK STRETCH

Perform 15 repetitions of this exercise.

EXERCISE 4
LAT PULL INS

Perform 12 repetitions on this exercise

EXERCISE 5
CHAIR DIPS

Perform 15 repetitions on this exercise

Rest for 2-3 minutes, then repeat these five exercises.

 Functional Movement 1

EXERCISE 1
CHAIR WARRIOR

EXERCISE 2
CHAIR REVERSE WARRIOR

EXERCISE 3
REVOLVED HEAD TO KNEE POSE

EXERCISE 4
SEATED WARRIOR II

EXERCISE 5
REVERSE TABLE TOP

Complete three sets of these 5 exercises, resting for 60 seconds between each set.

DAY 26 Core Strength

EXERCISE 1
CHAIR SPINAL TWIST

Do 15 repetitions of this exercise.

EXERCISE 2
CHAIR GODDESS TWIST

Do 15 repetitions of this exercise.

EXERCISE 3
CHAIR BOAT POSE

Do 12 repetitions of this exercise.

EXERCISE 4
MOUNTAIN CLIMBER

Do 15 repetitions of this exercise.

EXERCISE 5
PIKE PULSE

Rest for 2-3 minutes, then repeat these five exercises.

DAY 27 — Lower Body Strength

EXERCISE 1
LEG EXTENSION

Do 15 repetitions of this exercise on each leg.

EXERCISE 2
LEG DRAG

Do 15 repetitions of this exercise on each leg.

EXERCISE 3
LATERAL LEG LIFT

Do 15 repetitions of this exercise on each leg.

EXERCISE 4
SIT & STAND

Do 8 repetitions of this exercise.

EXERCISE 5
SEATED MOUNTAIN

Do 10 repetitions of this exercise.

Rest for 2-3 minutes, then repeat these four exercises.

EXERCISE 1
SEATED CHILD'S POSE

1. Sit upright in your chair with your feet flat on the floor.

2. Rest your elbows on your knees and lean forward to elongate your spine. Pull in your lower back and open your shoulder blades.

3. Now, extend your arms directly out before you, reaching forward to stretch the spine further.

4. Hold this position for 15 seconds.

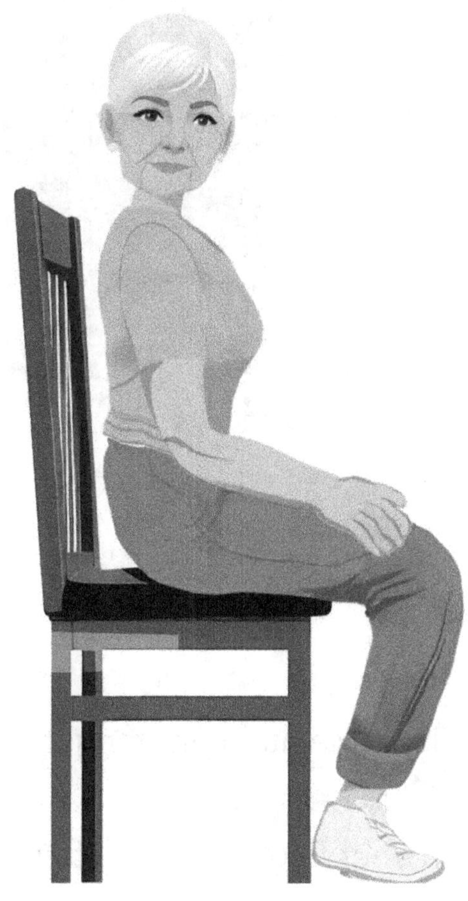

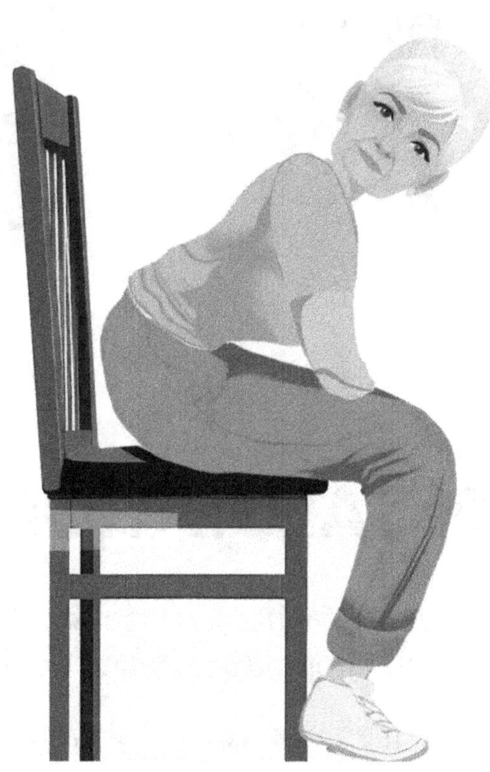

EXERCISE 2
SEATED PIGEON

1. Sit upright in your chair with your butt against the back support.

2. Bring your right ankle over your left knee.

3. Hold the ankle with both hands and gently draw it toward your body. Lengthen your spine and stretch your chest out as you breathe in and look toward the ceiling.

4. Hold this position for five deep breaths through your nose.

5. Repeat on the other side.

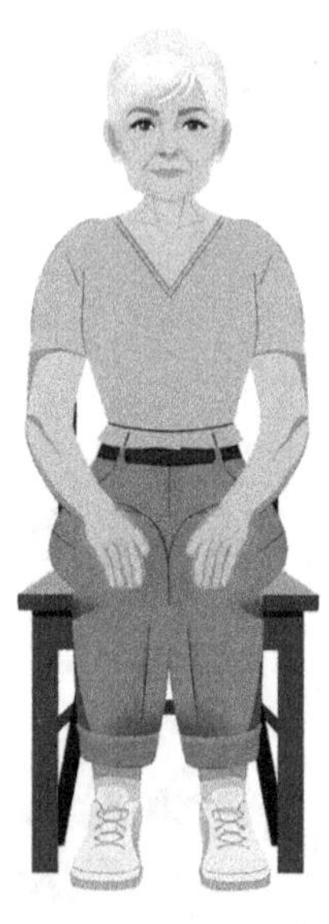
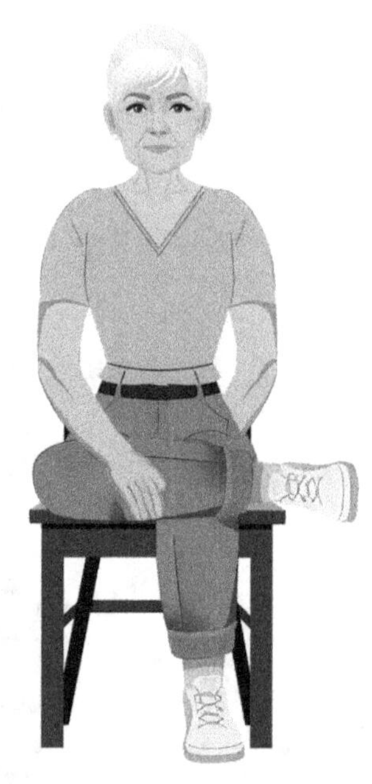
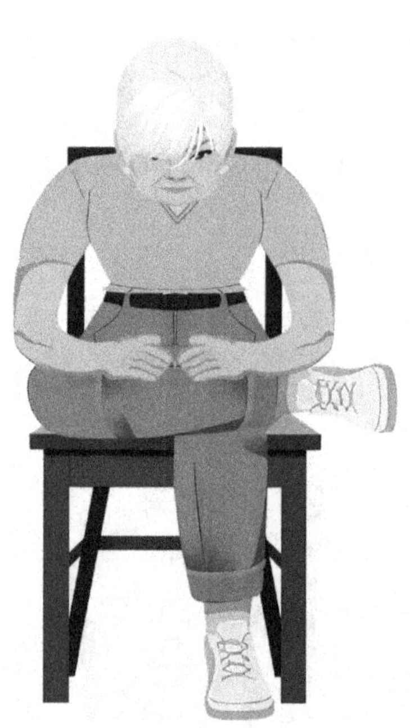

EXERCISE 3
SUN SALUTATION

1. 1. Sit upright with your feet firmly planted on the floor. Maintain an upright torso, with your shoulder blades pulled back and your chest open.

2. Inhale deeply as you reach your arms over to touch your fingertips together overhead.

3. Exhale as you lower your right arm and bend to the right side. Reach your left arm up and over your head as you feel the stretch through your right side.

4. Repeat on the other side.

5. Now, stretch your arms down as you bring your torso down and stretch forward.

6. Hold this position for 15 seconds.

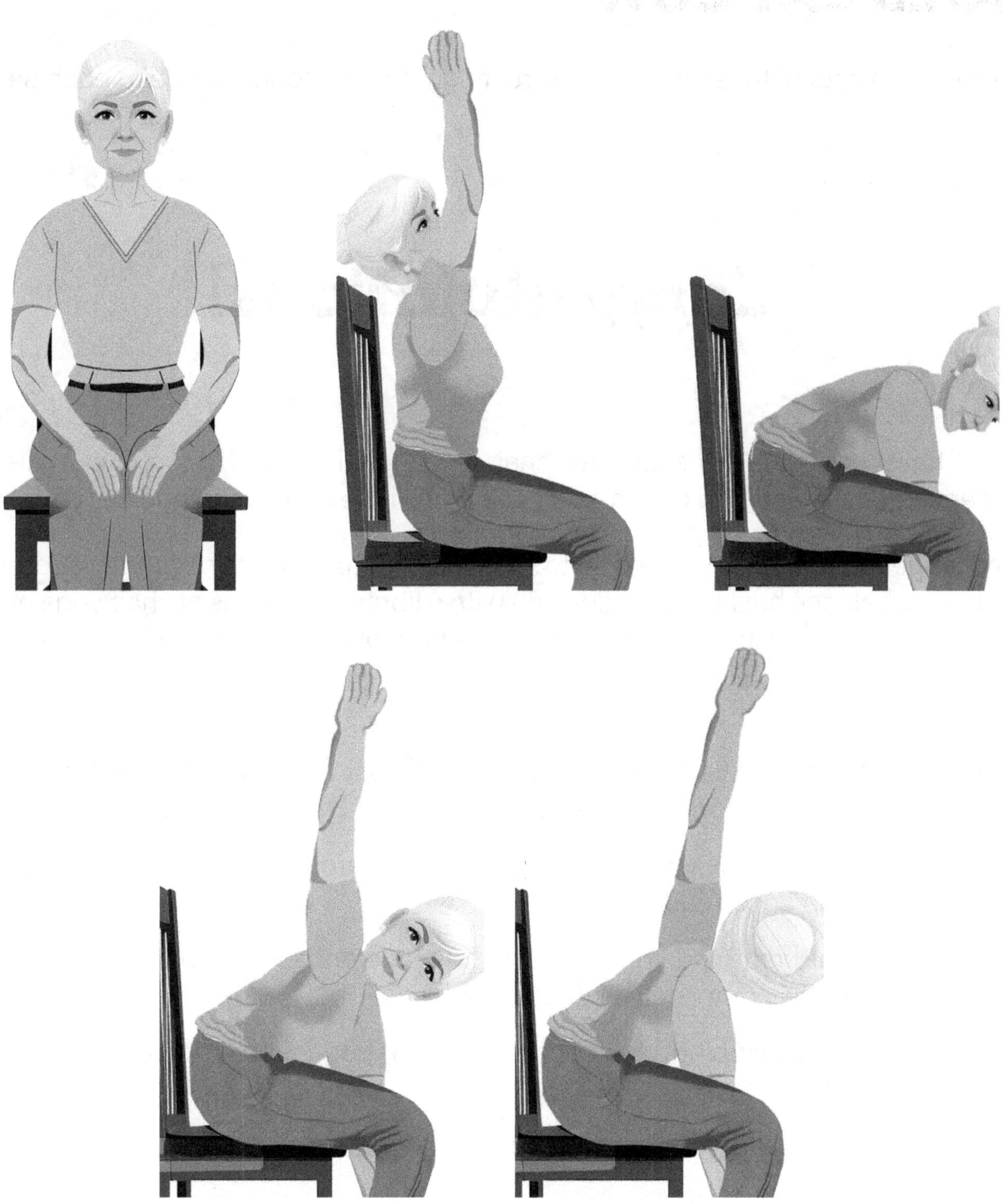

EXERCISE 4
BOAT POSE

EXERCISE 5
SEATED CAT COW

Complete three sets of these 5 exercises, resting for 60 seconds between each set.

Congratulations!

Your have completed the 28-day chair yoga challenge. Through your discipline, perseverance, and dedication, you have added the chair yoga habit to your lifestyle.

The challenge has not only allowed you to significantly improve your strength, coordination, flexibility, and balance but also provided you with a library of dozens of chair yoga exercises that you can use to construct your personalized workout going forward.

Here are some tips to help you do just that:

- Incorporate chair yoga into your daily routine. Just a few minutes each day is all you need to build upon the benefits you've gained from the 28-day challenge.

- Listen to your body as you perform your chair exercises. Stop if the exercise feels uncomfortable or painful.

- Focus on your breathing, remembering to inhale and exhale through your nose, filling your lungs completely with each breath.

- Stay hydrated by sipping from a water bottle before, during, and after your chair yoga sessions.

- Celebrate your success and embrace your newfound freedom and independence.

Healthy Meal Plan for Seniors Over 60

Eating for health is important at any age. But when you enter your sixties, maintaining a nutritious, balanced diet becomes more critical than ever. Our nutritional needs change as we grow older, requiring a focus on nutrient-dense foods that support overall health, energy levels, and vitality.

In this bonus section, we'll explore a sample healthy meal plan designed specifically for seniors over 60. The plan highlights essential nutrients and food groups to prioritize for optimal health.

BREAKFAST

Option 1: Oatmeal with Berries

Start your day with a bowl of oatmeal with raspberries, strawberries, or any other fresh berries. Oatmeal is a fiber-rich whole grain that provides sustained energy throughout the morning, while berries are packed with antioxidants and vitamins.

Option 2: Greek Yogurt Parfait

Enjoy a serving of Greek yogurt with sliced bananas, chopped nuts, and a drizzle of honey. Greek yogurt is high in protein, calcium, and probiotics, supporting bone health and digestive function. Nuts add healthy fats and crunch, while bananas provide potassium and natural sweetness.

Option 3: **Spinach and Mushroom Omelet**

Prepare a fluffy omelet with sautéed spinach, mushrooms, and diced tomatoes. Eggs are a rich source of protein and essential nutrients like vitamin D and B12, which are necessary for bone health and cognitive function. Spinach and mushrooms add fiber, vitamins, and minerals to this nutritious breakfast option.

MORNING SNACK

Option 1: **Mixed Nuts**

Enjoy a small handful of mixed nuts such as almonds, walnuts, and cashews as a mid-morning snack. Nuts are a great source of healthy fats, protein, and fiber, providing sustained energy and promoting heart health.

Option 2: **Fresh Fruit Salad**

Slice fresh fruits such as apples, oranges, and grapes to create a colorful fruit salad. Fruits are rich in vitamins, minerals, and antioxidants, supporting immune function and overall health. Enjoy the fruit salad alone or with a dollop of Greek yogurt for added protein.

LUNCH

Option 1: **Grilled Chicken Salad**

Prepare a hearty salad with grilled chicken breast, mixed greens, cherry tomatoes, cucumber slices, and avocado. Chicken is a lean source of protein, while vegetables provide fiber, vitamins, and minerals. Avocado adds healthy fats and creaminess to the salad, while a light vinaigrette dressing enhances flavor without excess calories.

Option 2: **Quinoa and Vegetable Stir-Fry**

Cook the quinoa following the instructions on the package, then stir-fry it with colorful vegetables such as bell peppers, broccoli, carrots, and snap peas. Quinoa is a complete protein and a good source of fiber, while vegetables add vitamins, minerals, and antioxidants. Season with soy sauce, garlic, and ginger for added flavor.

AFTERNOON SNACK

Option 1: **Hummus and Veggie Sticks**

Dip crunchy vegetable sticks such as carrots, celery, and bell peppers into creamy hummus for a satisfying and nutritious snack. Hummus is made from chickpeas, which are high in protein and fiber, while vegetables provide vitamins, minerals, and hydration.

Option 2: **Whole Grain Crackers with Cottage Cheese**

Enjoy a serving of whole-grain crackers topped with creamy cottage cheese for a protein-rich snack. Whole grain crackers provide fiber and complex carbohydrates, while cottage cheese is a good source of protein and calcium, supporting muscle health and bone density.

DINNER

Option 1: **Baked Salmon with Roasted Vegetables**

Bake salmon fillets seasoned with lemon juice, garlic, and herbs until tender and flaky. Serve with roasted vegetables such as Brussels sprouts, cauliflower, and sweet potatoes. Salmon is rich in omega-3 fatty acids, which support heart health and brain function, while vegetables provide fiber, vitamins, and antioxidants.

Option 2: **Vegetable Soup with Whole Grain Bread**

Prepare a hearty soup with seasonal vegetables such as carrots, celery, onions, and tomatoes. Add beans or lentils for extra protein and fiber. Serve with a slice of whole-grain bread for a satisfying and nutritious meal.

EVENING SNACK

Option 1: **Yogurt and Fruit Smoothie**

Blend Greek yogurt with your favorite fruits, such as berries, bananas, and mangoes, for a refreshing and nutritious smoothie. Greek yogurt provides protein and probiotics, while fruits add vitamins, minerals, and natural sweetness. Add a handful of spinach or kale for an extra boost of nutrients.

Option 2: **Whole Grain Crackers with Peanut Butter**

Enjoy a serving of whole-grain crackers spread with creamy peanut butter for a satisfying and protein-rich snack. Whole grain crackers provide fiber and complex carbohydrates, while peanut butter offers healthy fats, protein, and essential nutrients.

WRAP-UP

This sample healthy meal plan for seniors over 60 is designed to balance nutrients, including protein, fiber, vitamins, minerals, and healthy fats, to support overall health and well-being. By incorporating various nutrient-dense foods from all food groups, seniors can enjoy delicious and satisfying meals that promote energy, vitality, and longevity. Remember to stay hydrated throughout the day by drinking plenty of water and herbal teas and listen to your body's hunger and fullness cues to maintain a healthy relationship with food.

Healthy Habits for Weight Loss and Overall Health

Life is an accumulation of habits. If we can accrue more good habits and fewer bad ones, we will thrive physically and mentally. Here are eight wellness habits you should focus on and some tips on sticking with them.

#1: Establish a Bedtime Routine

Nothing will significantly impact your overall state of wellness more than the quantity and quality of your sleep. To get a great night's sleep each night, you need to establish a set routine. You can immediately do three things to make that happen...

1. Set a time to go to bed every night.

2. Turn your phone off 30 minutes before bed, and keep it out of your bedroom.

3. Develop a wind-down routine the hour before bed. You could include a warm bath, reading a book, or a period of mindful meditation.

#2: Eat Whole Food

Getting into the habit of eating real, whole food as close to its natural state as possible is a great habit. The key is to make small incremental changes. Here are three things you can do to develop the whole food habit...

1. Spend some time every Sunday preparing a large bowl of healthy, whole-food salad that you can keep in the fridge and serve throughout the week.

2. Start planning your meals for the week, accounting for times when you are on the run.

3. Experiment with a green smoothie to beat the mid-afternoon munchies.

#3: Practice Stress Release Habits

Many people are so busy that they never get time to pause and recharge, so it's hardly surprising that their stress levels are through the roof. You can't create more hours in the day, but you can spend a few minutes adding some habits to help you attain a calm state by de-stressing your mind and body. Here are three simple things you can start doing today...

- Stretch for 5 minutes with dynamic exercises that move your muscles through their full range of motion.

- Start journaling in the evening, recording your thoughts about your day.

- Go for a nature walk.

#4: Drink 2.25 Liters of Water Daily

Water is the elixir of life. It is amazing how much better your body and mind will function when you stay hydrated. Get into the habit of drinking 2.25 liters of water every day. You can do this by carrying a 750 ml bottle of water. Plan to get through it by 11 a.m. Then refill and drink consistently until 2 p.m. The final bottle should take you through dinner time.

#5: Eat More Slowly

Many people have developed the habit of shoveling food into their mouths, one spoonful after the other, without a break. It's as if they're racing to see who can finish eating first.

Generally, these people tend to have too much fat, whereas skinner people tend to eat more slowly. Let's find out why.

When you eat slower, you feel fuller faster. This is because your brain gets a chance to say, "I'm full," at a faster rate, as opposed to just shoveling the food in and ending up with a stomachache. To feel full, the brain must receive signals from hormones in the gastrointestinal tract.

Your stomach does not have teeth. So, everything that you put into it must be broken down. When you eat fast, your body doesn't have a chance to process the food. As you chew it in your mouth, saliva begins the digestive process. By the time it goes down your throat, a large part of the digestive process has already been accomplished.

But, when you swallow it down without chewing, you place undue stress on your gut. As a result, large pieces of unprocessed food can become trapped in the stomach, leading to gastric discomfort.

Get into the habit of chewing your food 10-15 times before swallowing. Put your fork down between mouthfuls. And engage in conversation while you're eating.

#6: Lift Weights to Lose Weight

Most people associate lifting weights with building muscles. Sure, they do that, but they also burn fat.

Exercising with weight resistance also releases the vital anabolic hormones testosterone and human growth hormone that promote fat loss. Recent studies indicate that, if done smartly, weight training can burn more calories than most forms of cardiovascular exercise.

Weight training will allow you to add muscle to your frame. Because muscle is so much denser than fat, a pound of muscle requires much more energy to sustain than a pound of fat. That means that every ounce of muscle you add to your body will increase your metabolic rate to burn more calories, even while at rest.

Contrary to what many women have been told, weight training does not make a person look bulky. Instead, it allows you to control the look of your muscles, sculpting a toned, tight, and lean physique.

#7: Fill Up on Fiber

Fiber is a form of carbohydrate that helps fill you, clean out your digestive system, and ward off hunger pangs. It also helps stabilize your blood glucose level, keeping your insulin level in check.

BEST FIBROUS CARB SOURCES

1. **Vegetables -** go for bright, colorful vegetables that are full of micronutrients

2. **Fruit -** choose such high-fiber fruits as berries (raspberries have 8 grams per cup), apples, peaches, oranges, and strawberries

3. **Beans, Lentils and Legumes**

#8: Meal Prep

Meal Prepping involves spending some time preparing your meals for the week, normally on the weekend. This makes it much easier for you to make healthy choices and far less likely that you will revert back to unhealthy eating habits.

Meal prepping will save you from having to cook at the end of the day. It will also help you avoid temptation when you're tired and hungry. That's because a nutritious meal will always be just a few minutes away. You'll save yourself from stressing out over food while saving money on your weekly food bill.

HOW TO DO MEAL PREP

- Set aside a definite time each week to do your prep – Sunday afternoon works well for many people.

- Write out your weekly menu, shop for the week, and then come home to get directly into the prep.

- Rely on staple food items that are easy to prep and cook.

- Start cooking your carbs first, as they generally take the longest

- Bake chicken breast, cook ground turkey, and make veggie patties, meatballs, etc.

- When you return from the supermarket, chop half of your veggies, then separate them into plastic bags. Chop the rest when you run out. You should also pre-make your salads and pre-chop the fruits that you will use for smoothies and snacks.

- Separate your meals into breakfast, lunch, dinner, and snacks daily.

- Store your food in the fridge in a Tupperware container or gallon zip-lock bag. Label each container with the day of the week that it is for.

Conclusion

Now that you've completed your 28-day chair yoga challenge acknowledge your incredible progress. You've shown determination, dedication, and resilience from the first day's tentative stretches to today's confident poses.

You've followed through on your commitment to show up in your chair each day. By doing so, you've chosen 28 times to prioritize your health and wellness. As a result, you'll now ingrained the chair yoga exercise habit into your lifestyle from now on.

That will only result in good things. Now, you can harness your renewed strength, balance, and mobility to live a more fulfilling, independent life.

But your journey doesn't end here; it's just the beginning of a lifelong practice of self-care that encompasses physical and mental rejuvenation.

So, as you close this book, take a moment to thank yourself for showing up, committing to your well-being, and embracing the journey. You are capable, you are strong, and you are enough. Keep shining bright and may your chair yoga practice continue to support and uplift you on your path.

Final Surprise Bonus

Hope you've enjoyed this *Chair Yoga for Weight Loss: 15-Minute Daily Exercises for Seniors Over 60 to Boost Strength, Flexibility, and Shed Pounds – Look and Feel Younger in Just 28 Days!*

We always like to give more than we get, so I'd like to give you one final bonus.

Do me a favor, if you enjoyed this book, please leave a review on Amazon.

If you do, I'll send you one of my most cherished Chair Yoga for Seniors Over 60 Workout Checklist – Free:

Chair Yoga for Seniors Over 60 Workout Checklist!

Here's how to claim your meal plan:

1. Leave a review right away –

2. Send a screenshot of your review to: reviews@idea2book.com with the subject line: " Chair Yoga for Seniors Over 60 Review"

3. Receive your – ***"Chair Yoga for Seniors Over 60 Workout Checklist!"*** – immediately!